CUPPING THERAPY
FOR BODYWORKERS

of related interest

Dry Needling for Manual Therapists
Points, Techniques and Treatments, Including
Electroacupuncture and Advanced Tendon Techniques
Giles Gyer, Jimmy Michael and Ben Tolson
ISBN 978 1 84819 255 3
eISBN 978 0 85701 202 9

Using the Bowen Technique to Address
Complex and Common Conditions
John Wilks and Isobel Knight
ISBN 978 1 84819 167 9
eISBN 978 0 85701 129 9

BodyMindCORE Work for the Movement Therapist
Leading Clients to CORE Breath and Awareness
Noah Karrasch with Robert White and Elizabeth Buri
ISBN 978 1 84819 338 3
eISBN 978 0 85701 295 1

CUPPING THERAPY FOR BODYWORKERS

A Practical Manual

ILKAY ZIHNI CHIRALI

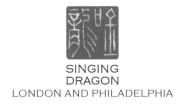

SINGING
DRAGON
LONDON AND PHILADELPHIA

First published in 2018
by Singing Dragon
an imprint of Jessica Kingsley Publishers
73 Collier Street
London N1 9BE, UK
and
400 Market Street, Suite 400
Philadelphia, PA 19106, USA

www.singingdragon.com

Copyright © Ilkay Zihni Chirali 2018

Library of Congress Cataloging in Publication Data
Names: Chirali, Ilkay Zihni, 1946- author.
Title: Cupping therapy for bodyworkers : a practical manual / Ilkay Chirali.
Description: London ; Philadelphia : Jessica Kingsley Publishers, 2018.
Identifiers: LCCN 2017060897 | ISBN 9781848193574 (pbk.)
Subjects: | MESH: Complementary Therapies--methods | Medicine, Chinese
Traditional--methods | Vacuum | Massage
Classification: LCC RM723.C5 | NLM WB 371 | DDC 615.8/220951-
-dc23 LC record available at https://lccn.loc.gov/2017060897

British Library Cataloguing in Publication Data
A CIP catalogue record for this book is available from the British Library

ISBN 978 1 84819 357 4
eISBN 978 0 85701 316 3

Printed and bound in Great Britain

*This book is dedicated to
Chanel, Ilkay and Yasmin.*

Acknowledgements

I wish to express my gratitude to all my patients who put their trust in me, and to all those who gave up their valuable time and volunteered for pictures to be taken for this book (Lisa Lewis, Hailey Westerman, Asim Dilaver, Maria Daly, Ilkay and Yasmin Hamit, Eddie and Nina Ertan). To my wife, Emine, who endured many solitary evenings while I was writing this book.

I would also like extend my sincere thanks to the publishing team at Singing Dragon, particularly to Claire Wilson, Senior Commissioning Editor, who prompted me to write this book.

Ilkay Zihni Chirali, 2018

Contents

Preface

For centuries, cupping therapy has been traditionally employed as one of the most effective and important tools of the Traditional Chinese Medicine arsenal.[1] As part of folklore medicine, too, many cultures from East to West and from North to South, over many thousands of years, have employed cupping therapy in order to treat a broad range of medical conditions, such as elevated blood pressure, the common cold and joint and musculoskeletal complaints, and to remove pus and infection from the body. Cupping was and still is used today in many Turkish baths (hamams) as a traditional relaxation medium as well as to treat painful and stiff joints and muscles.

Resurrection of cupping therapy

Internationally recognised personalities and celebrities, including Gwyneth Paltrow, David Beckham and, more recently, the swimmer Michael Phelps at the 2016 Rio Olympics, have candidly exhibited dramatic cupping marks on various parts of their body, leading to media frenzy! This has helped to reignite interest in this ancient but highly effective therapy, particularly from athletes, massage therapists and beauty therapists.

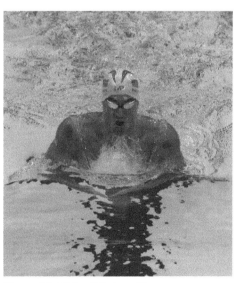

Figure P.1: Michael Phelps with cupping marks, at the Rio Olympics

1   Chirali, I.Z. (2014) *Traditional Chinese Medicine Cupping Therapy*, 3rd edition. Edinburgh: Churchill Livingstone.

While all this new interest in cupping therapy is taking place, many well-qualified people have taken up cupping practice; however, not-so-qualified people have also taken up cupping practices, offering cupping treatment in various locations, even on a kitchen table! As a devout cupping therapy practitioner and teacher, the issue of safe cupping practice is one of my main concerns. In recent years I have been called several times to act for litigation lawyers as a professional cupping therapy witness against cupping therapy malpractice in the UK. I sincerely hope that this book will give cupping therapists a clear and comprehensive guide and help contribute to safe cupping practice.

. . . .   ◆ ◆ ◆   . . . .

CHAPTER 1

A BRIEF HISTORY OF CUPPING

A personal journey

I was born in the village of Lemba (Çirali) near Paphos, Cyprus, where cupping was part of traditional Cypriot folklore medicine, practised by both the Turkish and the Greek population (Turkish – şişe düşürmek; Greek – ventouses). According to villagers, for the past two to three hundred years the accepted traditional practice was a cupping application for colds and coughs, and hemp tea for all other afflictions!

I experienced cupping on my body from a very young age and continue receiving it to this day. During my Traditional Chinese Medicine (TCM) studies in Melbourne, Australia, in the 1980s, I was lucky enough to have a teacher who also was a keen cupping therapy practitioner. Most acupuncture sessions at his TCM academy/clinic would conclude with a cupping treatment and Tuina (a TCM massage technique). In a short time, I found myself teaching cupping therapy techniques to new students at the college. I am a devoted cupping therapy practitioner and a teacher, and intend to continue to be so. For more than 35 years in a clinical environment, as well as outside clinical situations, I have witnessed first-hand the truly remarkable benefits of cupping therapy enjoyed by many men and women, old and young, particularly when their suffering was due to the common cold, asthma, pain and countless forms of muscular complaints.

Historical facts

This wonderful healing tool has been used by diverse traditional folklore practitioners for thousands of years. Cupping therapy is a universal practice and cannot be attributed to a single nation or tradition, but rather has spread in a vast geographical spectrum. From the warm Mediterranean villages of Cyprus to freezing towns of Sweden, and from isolated places in South America to modern towns in England, cupping is a familiar but often long-forgotten and 'out of fashion' medical practice. The doctors of ancient Egypt (around 3150 BC) were keen cupping practitioners, as the carvings of cupping equipment alongside various other medical instruments on the face of a temple in Luxor, Egypt clearly show. In traditional Jewish and Islamic (Hejama) medicine, too, cupping therapy has been extensively studied and practised throughout the ages. Hippocrates of Kos (400 BC), considered by many to be the founder of modern medicine, was a great advocate of cupping therapy in his teachings. The ancient Greeks and, later, the Ottoman Turks, who practised cupping in the traditional Turkish hamams, were mostly responsible for introducing cupping practices to the continent of Europe. From the 17th to the 19th century, cupping was extensively practised in all European hospitals, including in the UK, and in the USA.[1]

The Chinese Medicine doctors, however, are the true heroes who managed to keep the traditional methods of cupping practices alive and carried forward cupping knowledge as we know it today (**Figure 1.1**). Ancient cupping equipment comprised animal horns, clay cups, bamboo cups (still widely used today in Far Eastern countries) and porcelain cups. Glass cups were first used by the ancient Egyptians as early as 1500 BC. In Far Eastern countries, cupping therapy is still extensively practised, particularly during acupuncture and massage sessions. Throughout the 19th century many sophisticated manual and mechanical cupping machines were invented, particularly by American and European manufacturers.

Contemporary cupping therapy

As I am writing these pages today, in 2018, as far as the clinical practice of cupping therapy is concerned, we have truly come a long way!

....

1   Chirali, I.Z. (2014) *Traditional Chinese Medicine Cupping Therapy*, 3rd edition. Edinburgh: Churchill Livingstone.

....

Cupping therapy is no longer the exclusive tool of acupuncture practitioners. This ancient but effective treatment method has indeed managed to fascinate a broad range of healing professionals, resulting in much more extensive and sophisticated applications. *Cupping Therapy for Bodyworkers* is specifically intended for the non-Chinese Medicine practitioners, such as the sports physiotherapist, massage therapist and beauty therapist. It also gives directions on self-cupping application. Its purpose is to share my 50 years of cupping therapy experience and provide a clear, practical and detailed guide demonstrating how to administer cupping *safely and effectively*, in order to support practitioners in their own specialised field.

Figure 1.1: Chinese doctors practising/ teaching cupping therapy at China Medical University, Taichung, Taiwan

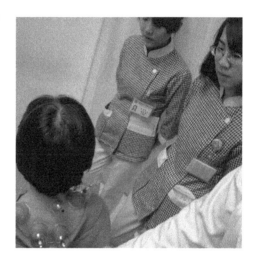

.... ◆ ◆ ◆ ....

CHAPTER 2

THE MECHANICS OF CUPPING THERAPY

How does cupping work?

Cupping works through the power of suction, which is created either by introducing a flame into the cup (this is by far the most popular method used in TCM clinics around the world) or by manually extracting the air from the cup (**Figures 2.1, 2.2**). The aim is to create a *controlled* vacuum within the cup. As a result, the skin and the fascia, in which the blood vessels, glands, nerves, muscles, ligaments and tendons are wrapped, are lifted and forcefully moved against atmospheric gravity towards the suction cup, resulting in local myofascial decompression. I have italicised the word 'controlled' in order to emphasise the importance of the need to control and manage the degree and intensity of the vacuum during the treatment, in order to avoid damaging the skin. This aspect of cupping therapy will be discussed time and again in the forthcoming chapters. The pulling action on the surface of the skin by the negative pressure inside the cup creates a movement that has a direct effect on both the superficial and the deeper levels of body fascia. This in turn leads to increased blood and fluid circulation, causing cellular, energetic and physical adjustments to take place, such as an increase in the metabolic rate. In my opinion, it is this conflicting gravity trick as well as the unexpected additional increase in micro-circulation that sends the self-healing mechanism into action!

Facing page:

Figure 2.1: Introducing a flame into the cup

Figure 2.2: Creating vacuum manually using a pistol-handled cupping set
One pull of the pistol handle creates a weak suction, two pulls a medium suction and three pulls a strong suction

....

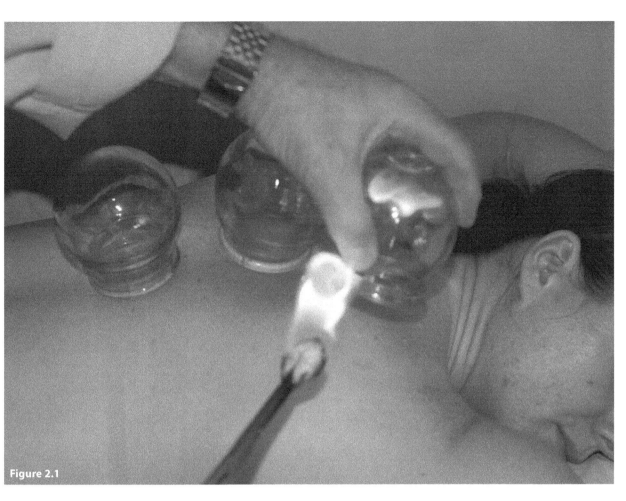

Figure 2.1

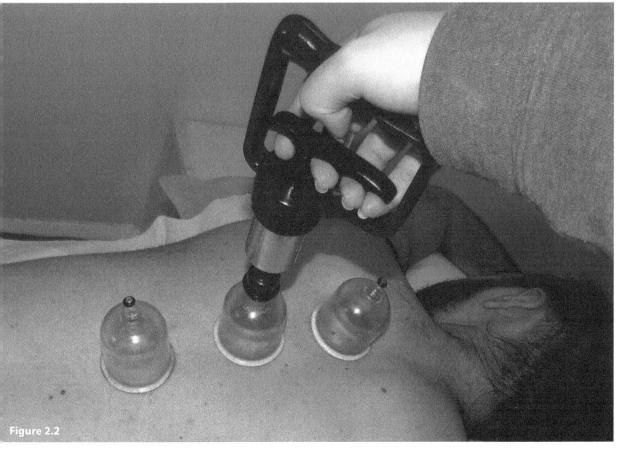

Figure 2.2

Cupping intensity

You will be surprised to discover the intensity and pulling power of the cup once the air is expelled from it! At all times during cupping application, any form of skin damage must be avoided.

Facing page:
Figure 2.3: Light cupping method
Minimal suction is created on the skin
Figure 2.4: Medium-strength cupping method
Moderate suction is created on the skin

- **Light cupping method:** With this method, the suction is minimal and the cup can move and slide on the surface of the skin effortlessly. Light cupping causes no significant marks on the skin. During the initial consultation and the first follow-up visit, I would strongly recommend the light cupping method. This is a safe way to introduce cupping suction on the skin (**Figure 2.3**).

- **Medium-strength cupping method:** With this technique, the suction is firmer and may leave cupping marks on the skin lasting up to ten days. Moving and sliding the cup on the surface of the skin requires moderate effort! Medium-strength cupping is the most frequently used cupping method of all. It is often employed during cupping massage applications (**Figure 2.4**).

- **Strong cupping method:** With this technique, the suction is really intense (**Figure 2.5**)! The skin and the fascia are pulled quite intensely towards the cup. Moving or sliding the cup over the surface of the skin is almost impossible and should not be attempted. This method is only applied as a static cupping method and should only be introduced following at least three light or medium-strength cupping applications to the same anatomical location. During strong cupping application, cupping marks are almost unavoidable and may last up to three weeks (**Figure 2.6**).

Benefits of cupping therapy

Skin

When it comes to skin nourishment and rejuvenation, cupping massage is probably the most effective natural therapy available. Here is why. Skin, the largest organ of our body, is the very first and most instantaneous beneficiary of cupping therapy application. This is where the initial contact is made by the suction cup and the chain of the stimulation process is set in motion. From here on, while performing cupping treatment, the cup and the skin become as one unit, intertwined. The feedback we are able to perceive through the skin, pre-treatment, during the treatment and post-treatment, is huge. The skin's reactions during the treatment – such as the colour, tightness or looseness, muscle tension, knots, pain, stiffness, cold, heat, sweat, dryness, lumps, bumps, scars, itching and relaxing – are the ongoing conditions that we can actually feel and experience just by gently touching the surface of the skin. Another interesting aspect of all of the above is that the manifestation of the disease and the treatment are both conveyed through

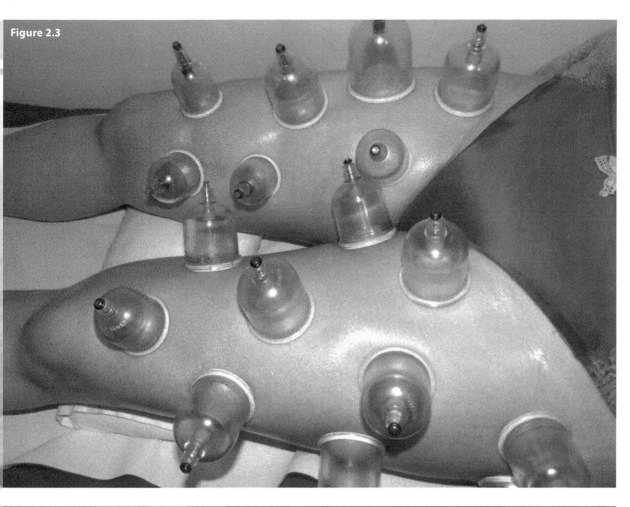

Figure 2.3

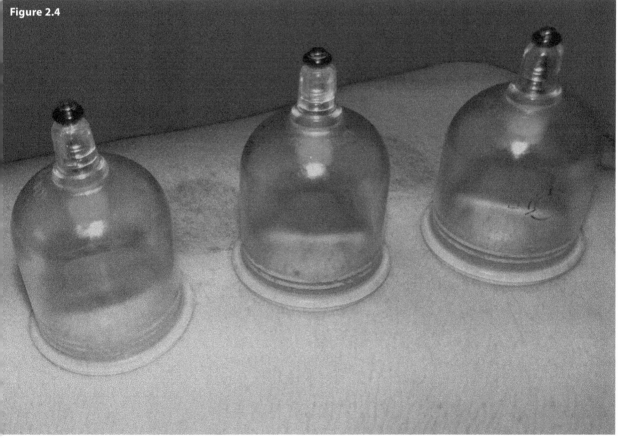

Figure 2.4

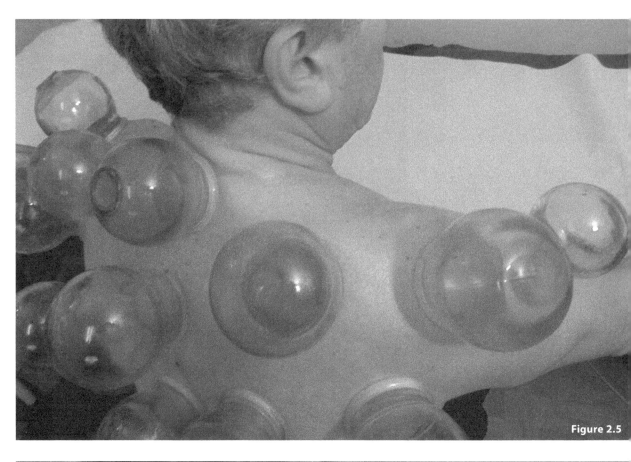

Figure 2.5

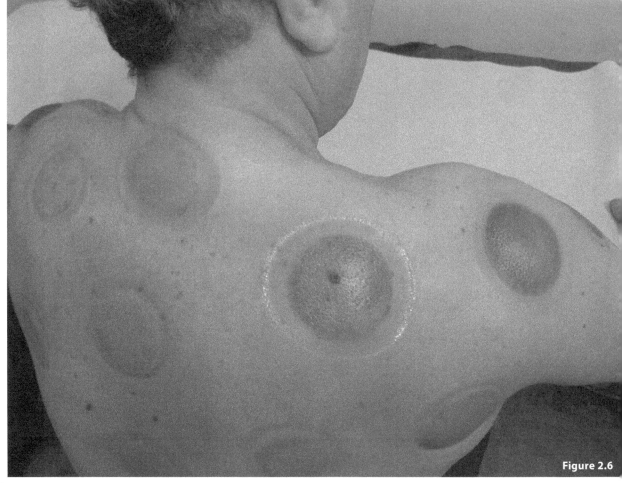

Figure 2.6

the skin. On the other hand, the prognosis – that is, the correct diagnosis and the cupping application technique that the practitioner will employ during the course of the treatment – will very much depend on his or her skill.

Fascia and muscle

Fascia is a jelly-like connective tissue made of collagen protein that attaches muscle to and separates it from internal organs. As described above, during cupping application the connective tissue fascia is simultaneously stimulated together with the skin. As a direct result of cupping application, the flow of oxygen-rich blood to muscle mass and the surrounding fascia is encouraged, resulting in improved muscle flexibility, stretching, muscle nourishment and energy surge to the treatment location.

Central nervous system

The next immediate beneficiary of cupping application is the central nervous system. Much like a complicated but very organised electrical wiring network in a large building, the human central nervous system is similarly responsible for transferring the external stimuli through the skin via the local skin receptors to the central nervous system (the feedback mechanism), to the brain and ultimately to the diseased organ. The interaction between the stimulation of the skin and the viscera (internal organs) is well documented by numerous scientific researchers. This intimate association between skin stimulation and the viscera is the key theory behind the cupping therapy function. A similar relationship in fact exists during an acupuncture treatment, namely the principle of meridians or channels, and the acupuncture points which are located on the fascia and their association with a particular organ and the central nervous system.

Body fluids and the circulatory system

From the very moment the suction cup engages on the skin, the local microcirculatory system is excited and invigorated. Depending on the dimension of the cup, each cup is capable of forcing a certain volume of blood and fluid to move towards the suction, resulting in hyperaemia (increase of blood flow in the vessels and body tissue). Cupping, no matter with what strength it is applied, promotes blood and fluid circulation by way of dilating and relaxing the blood vessels. This in turn helps to nourish and relax the muscle tissue, which can help with muscle performance and pain management (this is particularly effective when treating muscular pain, stiffness, joint pain, arthritis and neuralgic conditions). As therapists, we are all aware that for the healing mechanism to start functioning properly,

Facing page:
Figure 2.5: Strong cupping method
Skin is pulled quite forcefully into the cup
Figure 2.6: Cupping marks following strong cupping application

a fresh flow of oxygen-rich blood is necessary at the site of the affliction. I believe that cupping therapy is the perfect medium to do just that.

Immune system

As a direct result of increased microcirculation as described above, the lymphatic system is also excited and stimulated. The extra activity of the lymphatic system inevitably results in improved lymphatic drainage and the elimination of waste matter, reinforcing the entire immune system. These obvious physical benefits of cupping therapy unsurprisingly bring about mental and emotional respite, leaving the patient feeling uplifted and de-stressed. In countries such as China, Vietnam, Korea and Taiwan, it is quite common to see people walking in the streets bearing cupping marks on their body, especially prior to a season change. This is believed to give an extra boost to the immune system in order to increase the body's defence mechanism and protect the person from external pathogenic factors such as wind, cold, damp and heat.

A WORD OF CAUTION

Cupping therapy is strictly contraindicated for people who are currently receiving or have undergone any form of lymphatic cancer treatment, including surgery.

Safety: protecting yourself and the patient, and sterilising the cupping equipment

In order to avoid cross-infection, it is imperative that cupping equipment is sterilised after each use. One of the most effective ways to achieve 100% sterilisation is to bathe the cups in a 2% sodium hypochlorite solution after each use. With the wet cupping technique, however, after washing off the blood, it is more effective to leave the cups overnight in the sodium hypochlorite solution. It is better still to use disposable cups when administering the wet cupping technique. As far as the practitioner's safely is concerned, using an antibacterial handwash that contains a 20% chlorhexidine gluconate solution (Hibisol) between each patient not only provides the practitioner with effective protection against infection but is also considered to be good clinical practice.

Patient consent

It is also wise to ask the patient to sign a consent form. This is to confirm that you, as the practitioner, have explained the cupping procedure, the expectations, contraindications and especially the appearance of cupping marks on the skin. Depending on the patient's skin type, sometimes the cupping marks may last longer than expected. Almost all cupping marks will eventually clear completely without causing or leaving any permanent damage to the skin.

S A M P L E   C O N S E N T   F O R M

CUPPING THERAPY CONSENT FORM

I (patient's full name) . . . . declare that the cupping therapy practitioner (practitioner's full name) . . . . has fully explained to me the cupping therapy procedure, benefits, contraindications and possible side effects. I have been made aware that cupping marks may last between 8 and 20 days.

Signed . . . .

Date . . . .

.... ◆ ◆ ◆ ....

CHAPTER 3

CHOOSING THE RIGHT CUPPING EQUIPMENT

The enormous choice of cupping equipment offered on the market today can only be described as the cupping therapist's dream come true! As late as the 1990s, bamboo and glass cups were the only two types of cup available to cupping practitioners. Today, however, we are very fortunate to be able to choose from a large variety of cupping equipment.

Bamboo cups (Figure 3.1)

In the West, the bamboo cup is rarely used today. However, it is still very much favoured in Far Eastern countries. Bamboo cups are light enough to carry in a medical bag, especially when travelling to pay a home visit; they do not break easily and are quite inexpensive to buy. Nevertheless, there is one downside to bamboo cups: they cannot be fully sterilised due to the porous and absorbent nature of the bamboo itself. Therefore, it is not a very practical or safe choice in a busy clinic. The edges of bamboo cups can also dig into the skin during the application. This can be quite uncomfortable for some.

- Suction is created by briefly introducing a flame into the cup. The bigger the flame, the stronger the suction.

Glass cups (**Figure 3.2**)

Glass cups are by far the most popular type of cupping equipment used around the world today. Glass cups are easy to clean and sterilise, but they are expensive to buy and break easily when dropped. One of the most important advantages of the glass cup is that during the treatment the practitioner is able to observe and monitor the skin's reaction inside the cup, and take action accordingly – that is, remove the cup earlier if necessary.

- Suction is created by briefly introducing a flame into the cup. The bigger the flame, the stronger the suction.

Rubber cups (**Figure 3.3**)

Rubber cups are easy to use and clean, but expensive to buy. A disadvantage of the rubber cup is that in a short time (3–4 months) the massage oil used during the treatment tends to be absorbed by the rubber, destroying its quality and the smoothness of the cup's edges. This can cause unnecessary and avoidable discomfort when sliding the cup on the skin. Rubber cups are not suitable for the fire cupping technique.

- Suction is created by squeezing the air out of the cup and placing it on the skin. The more air is extracted, the stronger the suction becomes.

Silicon cups (**Figures 3.4, 3.5**)

Silicon cups are the latest variety introduced to the cupping family and are rapidly taking over from the more traditional glass cups. They are versatile during application, easy to clean, quite reasonably priced and come in all sorts of shapes and sizes. Silicon cups are not suitable for the fire cupping technique. Silicon cups are mostly favoured by the massage therapist and the beauty therapist. They are most suitable for sensitive parts of the skin and when cupping is performed on children or young adults.

- Suction is created by squeezing the air out of the cup and placing it on the skin. The more air is extracted, the stronger the suction becomes.

Manual and mechanical cupping equipment

This type of cupping equipment is manufactured either from glass or from a clear Perspex material. The pistol-handled cupping apparatus is one of the most popular types available (**Figure 3.6**). Air is extracted through a valve which is attached to the cup, or through an umbilical cord attached to a handle. Manual cupping sets have been around for many years, but the more sophisticated mechanical cupping equipment is relatively new to the cupping world. With mechanical cupping equipment, the air is extracted

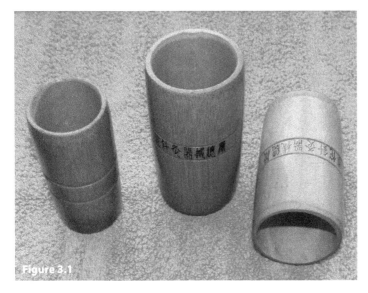

Figure 3.1

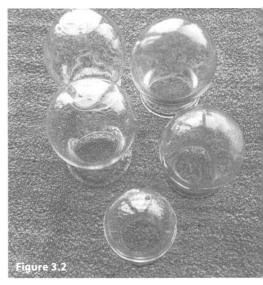

Figure 3.2

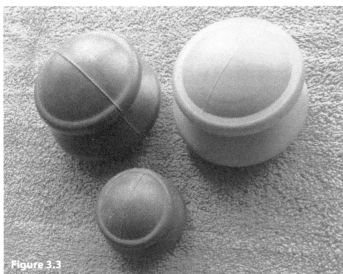

Figure 3.3

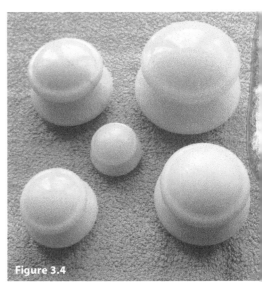

Figure 3.4

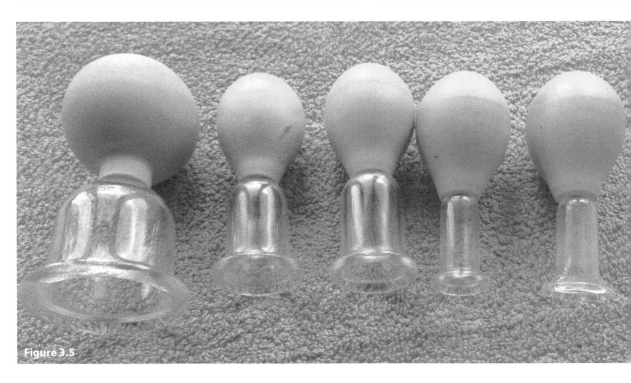

Figure 3.5

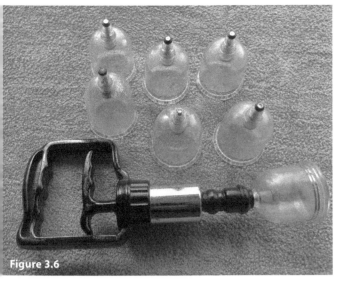

Figure 3.6

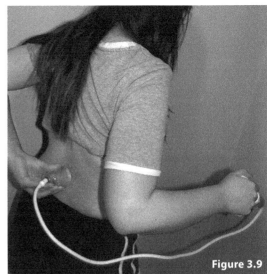

Figure 3.9

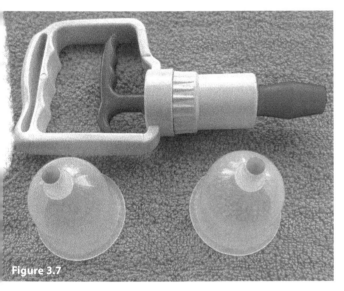

Figure 3.7

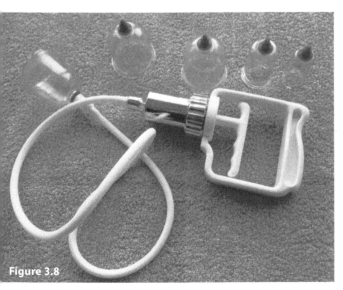

Figure 3.8

Facing page:
Figure 3.1: Bamboo cups
Figure 3.2: Glass cupping set
Figure 3.3: Rubber cups
Figures 3.4, 3.5: Selection of silicon cups
This page:
Figure 3.6: Pistol-handled cupping set
One of the most popular and practical cupping sets available
Figure 3.7: Disposable cupping set
Particularly valuable during bleeding (wet) cupping application
Figures 3.8, 3.9: Umbilical-corded cupping set
This cupping apparatus enables someone self-practising cupping to treat hard-to-reach areas of the body

by mechanical means. Some mechanical cupping equipment comes with additional features, such as being able to set the desired cupping time and suction strength. These types of cups are mostly favoured by the massage therapist and the beauty therapist.

- A single pull of the trigger provides light suction, two pulls provide medium-strength suction and three or more pulls provide strong suction on the skin.

Disposable cups for single use

Disposable cupping sets are the most recent variety introduced to the cupping practitioner. These are usually manufactured using a strong, clear recycled plastic material and are quite inexpensive to purchase. Disposable cupping sets are particularly useful when performing the bleeding (wet) cupping technique (**Figure 3.7**).

Umbilical-corded cupping set

The umbilical-corded cupping set has also been around for a number of years. This type of cupping set is mostly used during self-cupping application. The umbilical cord makes it possible to apply cupping to awkward and hard-to-reach locations on the body. The application is quite simple: using one hand, the person places the umbilical cup on the desired location and with the free hand pumps the air out of the cup, creating the desired suction. This type of cupping set is quite practical for self-cupping therapy, as the person applying the cups can determine both the strength and the timing of the treatment (**Figures 3.8, 3.9**).

.... ✦ ✦ ✦ ....

CHAPTER 4

CUPPING THERAPY TECHNIQUES

Cold cupping technique

When mechanical or manual cupping apparatus is used to achieve suction, the cupping application is described as 'cold cupping'.

Fire cupping technique

When a flame is used (no matter from what source) in order to achieve suction, the cupping method is termed 'fire cupping' or 'hot cupping'.

Before reaching for the flame, some patient and clinic preparation is necessary. The materials needed are: massage oil, cotton balls (preferably pre-soaked with pure alcohol and kept in an air-tight jar), long forceps, a lighter, numerous cups to be used during the treatment and a bowl of water to put the fire out after each use (**Figure 4.1**).

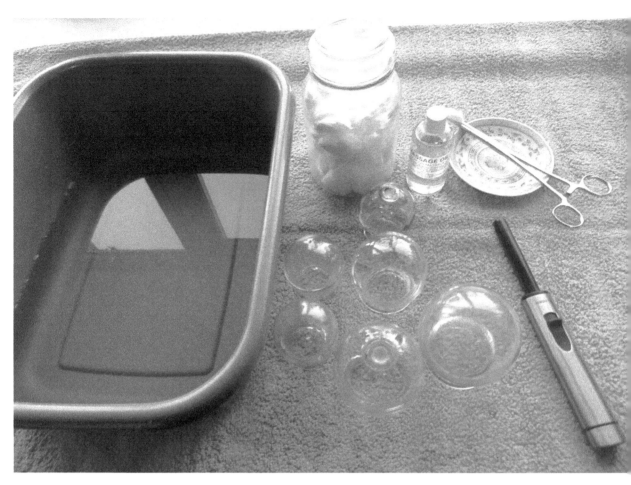

Figure 4.1: Equipment for fire cupping (cups of various sizes, alcohol-soaked cotton balls, long forceps, massage oil, lighter and water bowl)

Safe fire cupping application

Prepare your patient for massage in the normal way by removing clothing from the treatment location; remove all flammable materials around you and the patient, and make sure that the patient's hair is firmly secured. Apply massage oil liberally to the skin, and bring the cups to be used *close by the side of your patient* (**Figure 4.2**). By taking this precaution, you minimise the risk of dropping the lighted cotton wool on to the floor or, worse still, on to the patient! Secure a piece of cotton wool with the forceps and squeeze out the excess alcohol before lighting it (this will prevent burning alcohol dropping on bare skin) (**Figure 4.3**).

With your free hand, hold the cup upright; before inserting the flame fully into the cup, briefly hold the flame close to the cup edges to warm them – one or two seconds is usually sufficient (**Figure 4.4**). Once the edge is warmed, quickly insert the flame

Facing page:

Figure 4.2: Bring the treatment cups close to your patient

Figure 4.3: Secure the alcohol-soaked cotton wool using long forceps

Figure 4.4: Briefly warm the edges of the glass cups before placing them on the skin

Figure 4.5: Place the cup on the desired location

Figure 4.6: To reduce the strength of the suction or to remove the cup from the body, simply apply finger pressure to the edges of the cup in order to let air enter the cup

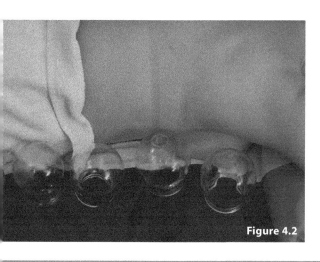

Figure 4.2

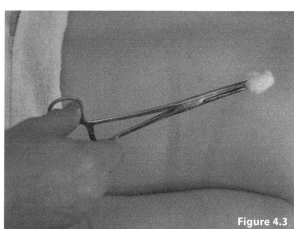

Figure 4.3

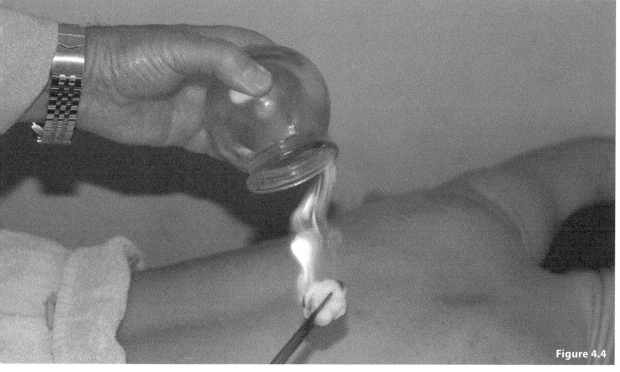

Figure 4.4

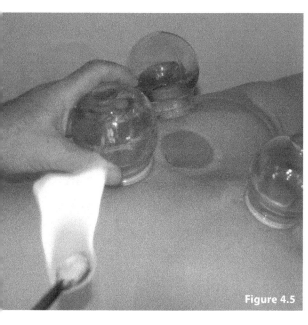

Figure 4.5

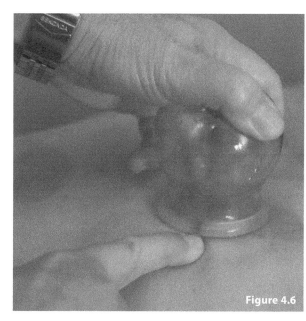

Figure 4.6

into the cup and then remove it. Then, without delay, place the cup on the bare skin at the desired location (**Figure 4.5**). Under normal circumstances, this will be adequate to achieve a firm suction. If the suction is excessive, which could cause discomfort or pain to the patient, the vacuum in the cup can be reduced by simply applying finger pressure between the skin and the cup, allowing a small amount of air into the cup (**Figure 4.6**). However, if the suction is too weak and does not hold the cup on the skin, this may be an indication of too much air remaining inside the cup. This is normally the result of a delay between inserting the flame and placing the cup on the skin. In this case, remove the cup and reapply, trying to be quicker this time. As with most things, the more you practise, the more proficient you will be.

The strength of the suction can also be adjusted as light, medium or strong (**Figure 4.7**). Light or medium-strength cupping is always preferred for the initial and second sessions of treatment. As the treatment progresses and if it is necessary, the strength of suction may be increased. During the treatment it is imperative that you communicate with your patient at all times, and provide reassurance if needed. With the light cupping technique, no significant cupping mark is left on the skin. With medium-strength cupping, a pinkish-red cupping mark is quite normal. With strong cupping, however, a dark red cupping mark can form quite rapidly. Also with the strong cupping method, if the cups are left in position for long periods of time (depending on skin type, this can vary between five and ten minutes), blisters can easily form on the skin. In order to avoid blisters forming, after applying the cups, stay with your patient and observe the reaction inside the cup. If there are any signs of blisters forming on the skin, remove the cup immediately and cover the blisters with a sterilised dressing. Refrain from cupping the same area until the skin is fully healed.

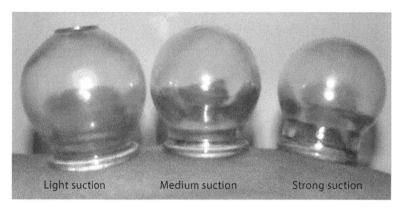

Light suction   Medium suction   Strong suction

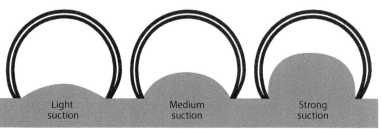

Light suction   Medium suction   Strong suction

Figure 4.7: The reaction of the skin and fascia inside the cup, showing light cupping, medium-strength cupping and strong cupping applications

CHAPTER 5

CUPPING APPLICATION VARIATIONS

No matter which type of cupping equipment is chosen during the treatment, different cupping techniques may be necessary to maximise the effectiveness of the therapy. The techniques listed below are the most frequently used variations during cupping therapy application.

Static cupping technique

In many folklore cupping practices, as well as in Traditional Chinese Medicine clinics around the world, the static cupping technique is by far the most practised cupping technique. A single cup or several cups are applied to predetermined locations and left in position for 3–15 minutes at a time. Static cupping can be achieved by all types of cupping equipment, but the most popular cupping equipment for this technique is the pistol-handled cupping pump. It enables the practitioner to be fast and in control of the situation at all times. This technique increases blood and fluid circulation, relaxes the fascia and helps to reduce inflammation and swelling, resulting in almost immediate pain relief (**Figure 5.1**).

Sliding cupping technique

The sliding cupping technique promotes blood microcirculation as well as lymphatic drainage, boosting the immune system and helping the process of eliminating foreign particles from the body. Sliding cupping is the most effective way to stimulate the dermal fibroblast cells which are responsible for the production of collagen and elastin proteins. Both proteins benefit the skin by giving strength and suppleness to the skin tissue. The sliding technique is mostly employed for dealing with skin toning, facial rejuvenation, water retention, oedema, lymph oedema, muscle stretching, muscle tightness, weight loss and cellulite complaints. For the cup to slide and move smoothly over the skin, the application of a generous amount of massage oil is always necessary. The movement of the cup should be smooth, with long and even strokes. Extra caution must be taken when treating people with sensitive skin. The sliding cupping method is mostly favoured by the massage therapist and beauty therapist (**Figure 5.2**).

Rapid cupping technique

The rapid cupping method is often employed as a warm-up technique, before the start of a more general cupping therapy session. This method is mostly applied to the entire back or the abdominal regions of the body. The rapid technique can be performed either with a single cup or with multiple cups. With the single cup method, the practitioner uses just one cup to apply and rapidly reapply the same cup to different parts of the body. With multiple cups, three or four cups are used at the same time. After applying all the cups on the body, the cups are immediately removed and reapplied in turn, starting with the first cup. The aim of rapid cupping is to warm the fascia and encourage microcirculation to a large section of the body (**Figure 5.3**).

Ice cupping technique

With the ice cupping method, prior to creating suction, one or two ice cubes are placed into the cup. Suction is achieved in the usual manner, either by inserting a flame into the cup or by mechanical means. After placing the cup on the skin, the cup must be continuously moved or rotated in short durations, lasting between five and ten minutes at a time and not exceeding 20 minutes in one session. The cup containing ice cubes must be moved continuously and not left standing on the same spot for any length of time. Ice touching bare skin can cause frostbite (ice burn), which can be as serious as the burn caused by a flame. This technique is mostly employed when treating muscular sprains, strains and inflammation, particularly when a heat pattern is accompanying the condition (**Figure 5.4**). (Patients with heat pattern usually complain of feeling hot and thirsty, have a red complexion and dry stools, are often restless and irritable and may experience sharp, stabbing pains. Conversely, patients with cold pattern complain of feeling cold and tired, are inactive and have a pale complexion often accompanied with dull muscular aches.)

Wet cupping (bleeding) technique

The wet or bleeding cupping technique is probably the oldest known cupping technique of all. The bleeding cupping method, alongside other bloodletting techniques, has been in practice for several centuries. Its main use was to purge the body of 'poisonous', 'unwanted' or 'foul matter'. During the 19th century a mechanical bleeding instrument called a 'scarificator' was invented in order to lacerate the skin (**Figure 5.5**). This bloodletting instrument was made of a matchbox-size unit, which contained six or more blades attached to a rotating lever. The practitioner would place the box on top of a desired location and with a flick of the lever the blades would rotate and cause a superficial laceration on the skin, about 1cm long and 3mm deep. The practitioner would then proceed to place a suction cup over the incision and extract blood into the cup. The amount of blood drawn would vary between 20ml and 100ml (depending on the cup size and the cupping duration).

In today's modern clinics, wet cupping is performed by using disposable needles or a surgical lancet. Careful planning is also needed before and after the treatment. There are two ways of performing a wet cupping treatment.

(1) Begin by sterilising the area to be treated with a sterilising solution. Using a surgical lancet or a needle, prick the skin to bleed. If a surgical lancet is used, the cut should be superficial and no bigger than 1cm long and 3mm deep. Once the bleeding is achieved, place a large suction cup over the cut. In a short time you will observe blood running into the cup. Carefully remove the cup once the desired amount of blood has been extracted. During the removal of the cup, spillage of blood can be avoided by holding an additional towel under the cup. A sitting-up position is usually preferred during a wet cupping application.

(2) For the second wet cupping method, first, in order to force blood flow to the surface of the skin, a regular dry cup is applied to the treatment area for ten minutes and then removed. The treatment area is sterilised and bled by a single cut or several tiny cuts. Once the area is bleeding, a large suction cup is placed over the incision and the blood flows freely into the cup. When the desired bleeding is achieved, the cup is removed by holding it firmly with one hand, while the other hand slides and lifts the cup from its place. Sterilise the area once more and cover with a gauze dressing.

The wet cupping method is administered in order to disperse blood stagnation and promote fresh blood circulation to the targeted site. When the body is bled, this sets off a chain reaction which triggers the bone marrow to regenerate new erythrocytes

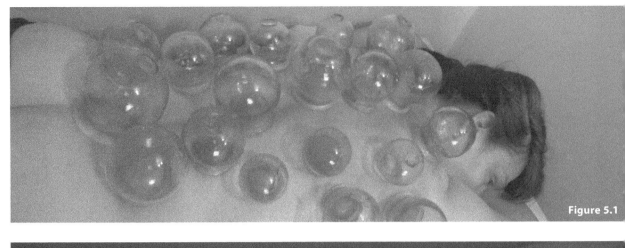

Figure 5.1

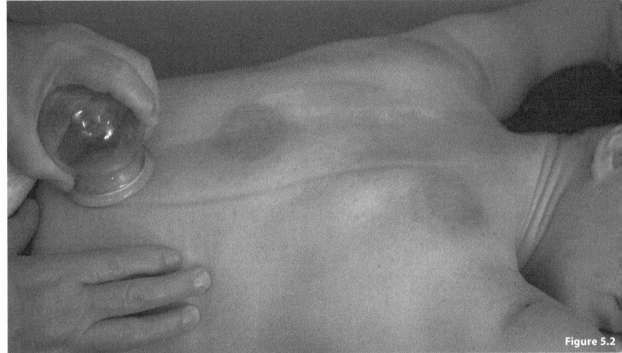

Figure 5.2

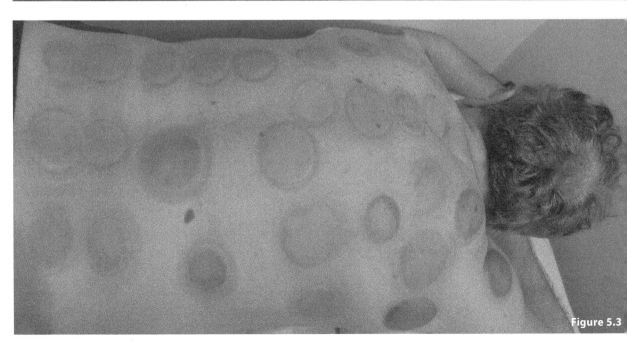

Figure 5.3

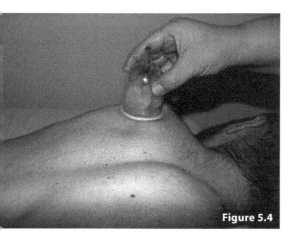

Figure 5.4

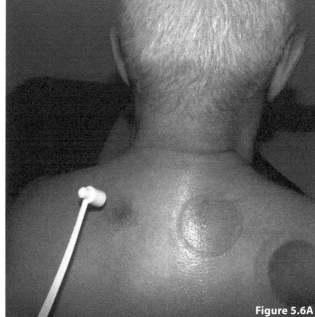

Figure 5.6A

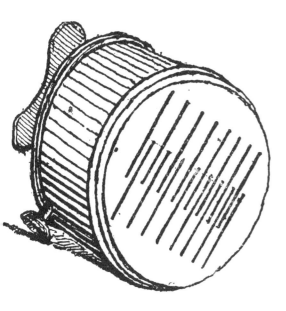

Figure 5.5

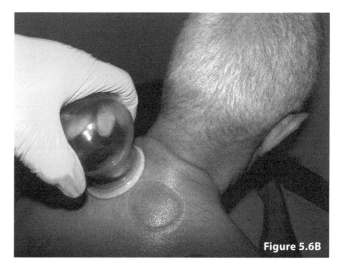

Figure 5.6B

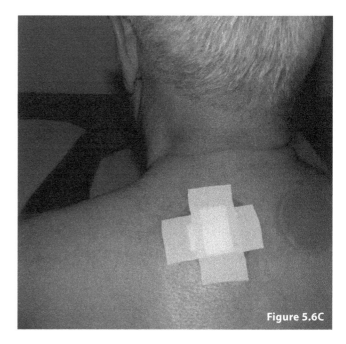

Figure 5.6C

(red blood cells) and an increase in leucocytes (white blood cells). Following bleeding, local blood pressure is also reduced, allowing normal blood flow to resume. This technique is particularly effective when dealing with sports injuries and chronic joint problems accompanied by a heat pattern. Disposable cupping sets are now available specifically for use in wet cupping applications (**Figure 5.6A, B, C**).

Hot or cold cupping therapy?

I am often asked which type of cupping therapy is more effective – the hot/fire cupping method or the cold cupping application.

Both cupping methods are equally effective! The application type will depend very much on the patient's condition. On most healthy individuals, both methods can be applied to maximum effect. However, if a patient appears to be suffering from any form of cold pattern – such as generally feeling cold, the common cold, trembling or feeling cold when palpated – the hot cupping method should always be preferred over the cold application. Equally, if an obvious inflammation is present at the treatment location, then the cold cupping method will be the more appropriate choice.

.... ♦ ♦ ♦ ....

CHAPTER 6

WHAT TO ANTICIPATE DURING CUPPING THERAPY

Each body massage or manipulation method has its own signature technique. Where some methods have gentle touch and smooth movement on the skin surface, other techniques require stronger pressure or even 'digging' techniques on the skin's surface. All massage techniques are designed to encourage lymphatic drainage and blood circulation, undo muscular tension and bring a sense of well-being and relaxation to the recipient.

With cupping therapy, however, the unique feeling is one of a 'pulling' sensation on the skin surface where the cup is actually engaged. During a cupping session, healthy skin is expected to react by becoming warm and turning a slightly pinkish-red colour. Therefore, the skin's reaction also becomes an important part of the diagnosis process! If the colour of the skin remains unchanged, this could be an indication of poor blood circulation or a cold pattern present at the treatment location. The significance of skin colour changes during a cupping session is explained in the following section.

Under normal circumstances, the patient should not experience any pain at all, but rather a mild, medium or strong pulling sensation (depending on the type of treatment method being employed). Post-treatment, most patients report a sense of warmth, relaxation and uplifting. Feeling light-headed is also quite common. This is due to an increased blood flow to the brain. Therefore, following a cupping session, it is considered good practice to allow a few minutes' rest and a warm drink before the patient leaves the clinic.

What is in the colour?

Typically, on the first and second sessions of the cupping treatment, it is quite normal to see an exaggerated skin colour (pink or red cupping marks) appearing on the cupped location. These cupping marks usually clear within ten days. However, depending on the skin type, dark red or purple cupping marks could take up to two weeks or longer to clear completely (**Figure 6.1**).

How to interpret the colour of the cupping marks diagnostically is explained below and in **Figure 6.2**.

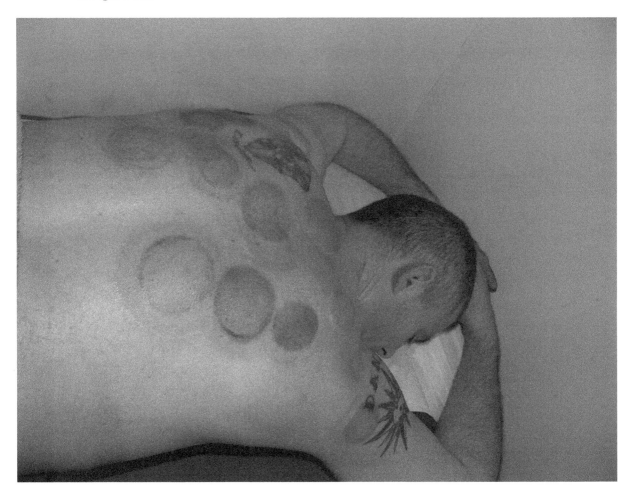

Figure 6.1: Excessive cupping marks on the skin may last several weeks

- **Pink to light red:** This is the expected colour for healthy skin to appear immediately following the treatment. It is an indication of good blood supply and circulation at the treatment location.

- **Bright red:** Bright red cupping marks on the first and the second visit are considered normal cupping marks. However, longer-lasting (more than a week) bright red cupping marks may indicate a possible inflammation or some level of blood stagnation. As a rule, long-lasting bright red skin colour at the site of cupping indicates blood stagnation. This is often seen during the treatment of chronic muscular tension, tightness, trauma or sports injuries.

- **Dull red:** This may be an indication of a chronic injury or a blow to the location.

- **Dark red or purple:** Dark red or purple cupping marks are a sign of a chronic blood stagnation or toxin build-up at the treatment site. This is the aspect of cupping therapy most disliked by patients. As the treatment progresses, however, the intensity of the colour is reduced. This also suggests a reduction of the blood stasis or elimination of toxins, leading to a normal blood flow and lighter cupping marks. Failure to adjust the cupping duration or intensity of the suction is the main cause of excessive blood flow to the skin tissue, which can cause dark red or purple skin colour or blisters to form on the skin. These extreme cupping marks are sometimes referred to as extravasates or haematomas. Recent trauma is another factor. However, when these extravasates or haematomas completely clear, there is rarely any permanent damage to the skin.

- **Pale:** Pale skin colour at the treatment site could be an indication of poor blood supply, inadequate blood circulation or a cold pattern present at the treatment location. This is often seen in people working outdoors and complaining from lower back pain. Usually, cold and wind penetrate the skin into the deeper muscular layers, causing stricture in blood vessels and resulting in poor blood circulation that can lead to muscle spasm and pain. However, as the treatment progresses, the usual healthy pink-red skin colour should return (this may take between six and ten visits).

- ⬤ *Pink to light red: indication of normal blood flow to the treatment location*
- ⬤ *Bright red: indication of possible local inflammation*
- ⬤ *Dull red: indication of chronic blood stagnation*
- ⬤ *Dark red or purple: indication of 'cold pattern' accompanied by blood stagnation or build-up of toxins*
- ⬤ *Pale: indication of 'cold pattern' or poor blood circulation at the treatment location*

Figure 6.2: Significance of the cupping marks on the skin

CHAPTER 7

CUPPING THERAPY FOR ATHLETES

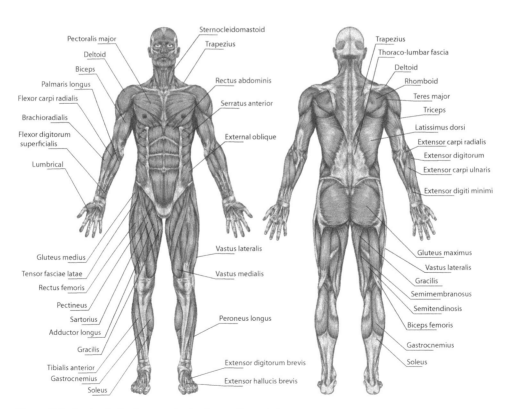

Figure 7.1: Anatomical reference chart   *Source: Shutterstock*

Effects on muscle performance

Let's take a closer look at the basic function of the muscle tissue. Muscles are strong fibrous tissues which are responsible for all bodily movements. They also contain abundant blood vessels and nerves. Every bodily movement, however insignificant, is made possible by muscles and tendons. Muscles work in a group rather than individually. Every skeletal movement is enabled not by a single muscle but by a group of muscles. Broadly speaking, muscles in human anatomy are classified into three groups. First is the voluntary muscle, also called 'skeletal muscle', which we are able to control, such as hand, leg and neck muscles. Voluntary muscles are distributed throughout the body. Second is the involuntary muscle, also called the 'smooth muscle', which we are not able to control, such as the gut and bladder muscles. Third is the cardiac muscle (heart muscle).

To function properly and generate energy, all muscle types need the same ingredients: (1) fuel, in the form of blood, in order to supply the muscle with oxygen and nutrients such as vitamins and minerals, and (2) efficient lymphatic drainage, to facilitate the disposal of waste resulting from muscle metabolism. Strong and healthy muscle should have good blood supply; flexibility, with the capability to quickly stretch and rapidly return to its original state; and no area of pain, stiffness or adhesions.

Sometimes athletes put too much emphasis on muscle-building programmes and the physique, rather than working on the total health of the body itself! Muscle injury and muscle fatigue are often the result of overuse. Exercising muscle excessively leads to oxygen depletion and the build-up of waste in the form of lactic acid. Both conditions can manifest as muscular pain, muscular cramps, stiffness, adhesion, tiredness, under-performance or delay in recovery. Over-exercise can also tax the heart and the kidneys.[1]

Cupping therapy during rehabilitation programmes

Cupping therapy is an excellent treatment for reducing muscle recovery time following an injury or over-exercise. According to Assistant Clinical Professor of Orthopaedic Surgery, Giles R. Scuderi, MD, the co-author of *Sports Medicine*, 'Local tissue oxygenation (pO2, tissue partial pressure of oxygen) is the single most important factor in wound healing.'[2] Most sports physicians also agree that muscle recovery takes place during resting, and not while exercising. To maximise muscle recovery, a period of rest and a gentle stretching protocol to promote blood and fluid circulation is essential. During this phase, light or medium-strength cupping is the perfect treatment to encourage the fresh flow of oxygen and nutrients to tired or injured muscle mass in order to shorten recovery time.

1   Barach, J.H. (1913) *Against Over-Athleticism.* From the Transactions of the Fourth International Congress on School Hygiene, Buffalo, NY, August 1913.

2   Scuderi, G. and McCann, P. (2004) *Sports Medicine: A Comprehensive Approach*, 2nd edition. Philadelphia, PA: Elsevier Mosby.

Cupping therapy application to skeletal muscles:

- triggers the rapid flow of oxygen-rich blood and nutrients to muscle tissue, thus increasing muscle performance and promoting the healing of tissue damage

- improves circulation of blood and lymph by eliminating tissue fluid beneath the skin

- increases tissue elasticity and reduces muscle tightness

- assists with the flow of nutrients to muscle and bones

- leads to oxygen saturation in the superficial muscular mass

- relaxes muscle and tendons

- relieves muscular tension and pain

- softens and helps stretch the muscle fibres

- increases the flexibility and strength of muscle

- improves joint mobility and muscular flexibility

- benefits joints by relieving excessive muscle tension

- helps to reduce muscular adhesion

- helps restore muscle tone

- benefits lymphatic circulation of the skeletal muscle and assists with the elimination of waste matter

- brings energy to muscles and helps shorten the recovery cycle, particularly during the rehabilitation period.

Sports performance and cupping therapy protocol

Start the cupping application by employing light to medium-strength static cupping, initially lasting 5–10 minutes, increasing the duration as well as the suction strength during follow-up visits. After removing the static cups, continue with the cupping massage application, employing the sliding cupping technique. Following the contour of the muscles during the cupping application is the most effective method when dealing with muscular complaints. For muscle injuries such as strain, sprain, tendinitis and restricted joint movement, apply the same treatment protocol.

Depending on the complaint or the condition, the frequency of cupping can vary between one and three times per week. Generally speaking, the more chronic the condition, the more treatment may be necessary. In the event of muscular or joint inflammation, employ the ice

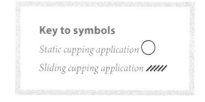

Key to symbols
Static cupping application ◯
Sliding cupping application ⫽⫽⫽⫽

cupping technique using light or medium-strength cupping application. Avoid cupping on a recent injury, trauma or contusion.

In this section I'll outline the benefits that cupping therapy can bring athletes in the following sports – before, during and after they take part in the particular sporting activity.

- Archery

- Bat- and club-based sports (baseball, cricket, golf)

- Cycling

- Darts

- Discus

- Football

- Net-based sports (baseball, netball, volleyball)

- Racket-based sports (badminton, squash, table tennis, tennis)

- Running

- Ski-based sports (skiing, waterskiing)

- Swimming

- Water sports (rowing, kayaking, canoeing, sailing, white water rafting, sculling)

- Weightlifting and powerlifting

For easy reference I have included charts identifying the muscle groups and possible injury sites, as well as the cupping application locations, for each type of athlete.

Archery

ANATOMY INVOLVED

Archery is a non-contact sport that does not normally expose the body to a lot of injuries. It is less energetic compared with most other sports. However, the repetitive movement involved in practice and competition does put the archer at risk for repetitive strain injury (RSI). It is advised that archers should use regular strength and flexibility exercise to offset overuse injuries from the repetitive actions. Although the stress is on the upper body, strong leg muscles provide a solid foundation for the shot.[3]

MAIN MUSCLE GROUPS USED IN ARCHERY

- The muscles of the shoulder girdle: the latissimus dorsi, the teres major and the deltoids.

- The muscles of the neck: the levator scapula and trapezius muscles.

- The core muscles: the rectus abdominis, obliques and spinal erectors.

- The muscles of the upper legs and hips: the gluteals, the hamstrings and the quadriceps.[4]

MOST COMMON ARCHERY INJURIES

- Rotator cuff injuries (see **Figure 7.3**).

- Tendinitis.

- Muscle strains.

- Contusion.[5]

....

3   Haywood. K.M. and Lewis, C.F. (1997) *Archery: Steps to Success*, 2nd edition. Champaign, IL: Human Kinetics Publishers.

4   Walker, B. (2017) 'Archery stretches and flexibility exercises', StretchCoach website, http://stretchcoach. com/articles/stretches-for-archery

5   Walker, B. (2017) 'Archery stretches and flexibility exercises', StretchCoach website, http://stretchcoach. com/articles/stretches-for-archery

....

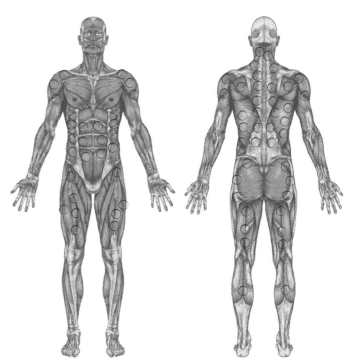

Figure 7.2: Potential archery injuries and cupping therapy locations

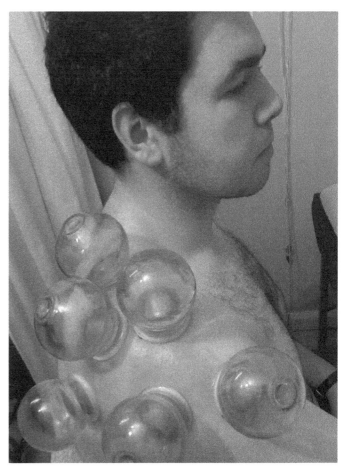

Figure 7.3: Treating a rotator cuff injury with cupping therapy
Rotator cuff injury is one of the most frequently seen sports injuries at the clinic

Bat- and club-based sports (baseball, cricket, golf)

ANATOMY INVOLVED

Bat- and club-based sports such as baseball, cricket and golf put a lot of stress on the upper limbs, particularly the shoulders, elbows and hands.[6] The action of throwing begins at the feet and ends at the fingers of the throwing arm, forming a kinetic chain of events that must link together in a specific way for optimal performance. A kinetic chain is defined as 'a coordinated sequencing of activation, mobilisation, and stabilisation of body segments to produce a dynamic activity'.[7]

MAIN MUSCLE GROUPS USED IN BAT- AND CLUB-BASED SPORTS

- The front and back muscles of the upper torso: sternocleidomastoid, deltoids, pectorals, trapezius, triceps, biceps, the abdominals, latissimus dorsi and erector spinae.

- Leg muscles: the hamstrings and quadriceps.

- The forearm muscles: the extensors and flexor muscles.

MOST COMMON BAT- AND CLUB-BASED SPORTS INJURIES

- Head and face.

- Neck, spine and back.

- Shoulder and chest.

- Arm and elbow (see **Figure 7.5**).

- Wrist, hand and fingers.

- Abdomen, hip and groin.

- Upper leg.

- Knee.

- Ankle, foot and toes.[8]

6   British Medical Association (2010) *The BMA Guide to Sports Injuries*. London: Dorling Kindersley.

7   Mallac, C., The Sports Injury Doctor website, www.sportsinjurybulletin.com, Bulletin No. 130.

8   British Medical Association (2010) *The BMA Guide to Sports Injuries*. London: Dorling Kindersley.

Bat- and club-based sports
(baseball, cricket, golf)

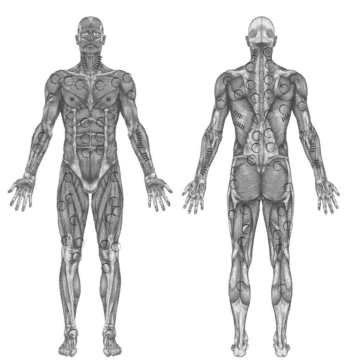

Figure 7.4: Potential bat- and club-based sports injuries and cupping therapy locations

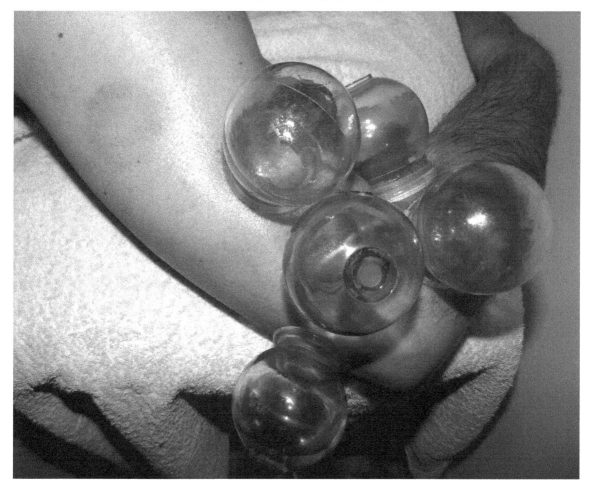

Figure 7.5: Treating 'golfer's elbow' syndrome

Cycling

ANATOMY INVOLVED

Cycling is considered to be a 'low-impact and weight-bearing sport activity'[9] that can be performed by young people as well as individuals past their 70s! When riding a bike, all body muscle groups are activated. Lean, flexible and strong muscle structure is advantageous. 'Cycling fitness is determined largely by strength, cardiovascular endurance, muscle endurance, and power.'[10]

MAIN MUSCLE GROUPS USED IN CYCLING

- The upper body (shoulder, chest and arms): pectoralis major, deltoids, biceps and triceps.
- The lower body: the gluteals, hamstrings, quadriceps and gastrocnemius.

MOST COMMON CYCLING INJURIES

- Neck, spine and back.
- Shoulder and chest.
- Arm and elbow.
- Wrist, hand and fingers.
- Upper leg.
- Knee (see **Figure 7.7**).
- Lower leg.
- Ankle, foot and toes.[11]

9   Andrews, G. and Doughty, S. (2007) *The Cyclist's Training Manual*. London: A&C Black.

10   Laurita, J. (2013) *Anatomy of Cycling*. London: Bloomsbury, p.11.

11   British Medical Association (2010) *The BMA Guide to Sports Injuries*. London: Dorling Kindersley.

Cycling

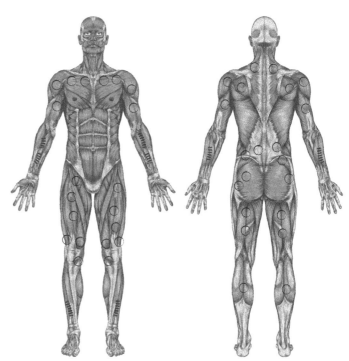

Figure 7.6: Potential cycling injuries and cupping therapy locations

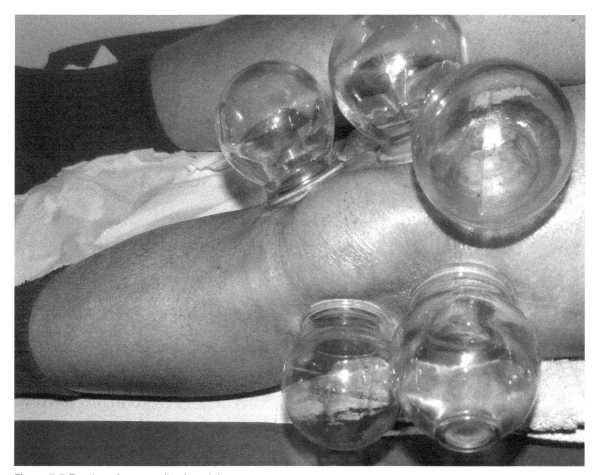

Figure 7.7: Treating a long-standing knee injury
Knee injury is another frequently seen condition at the clinic

Darts

ANATOMY INVOLVED

A game of darts is mostly played casually in pubs by young and not so young, male and female players. It can be a relaxing game but also a competitive sport. No matter how it is played, strong arm muscles, flexibility and good eye-to-hand coordination are essential requirements during a game of darts.

MAIN MUSCLE GROUPS USED IN THROWING A DART

- The shoulders: trapezius, deltoids and the rotator cuff muscles.
- Upper arm muscles: the biceps and triceps.
- Elbow, forearm and wrist: the hand extensors and flexors.

MOST COMMON DART-THROWING INJURIES

- Shoulders.
- Neck (see **Figure 7.9**).
- Elbow.
- Forearm.
- Wrist.

Darts

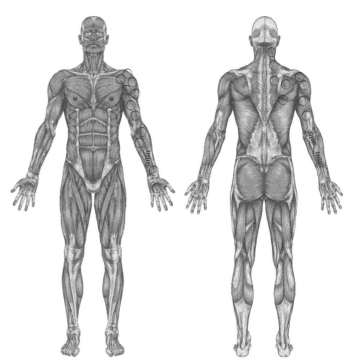

Figure 7.8: Potential dart-throwing injuries and cupping therapy locations

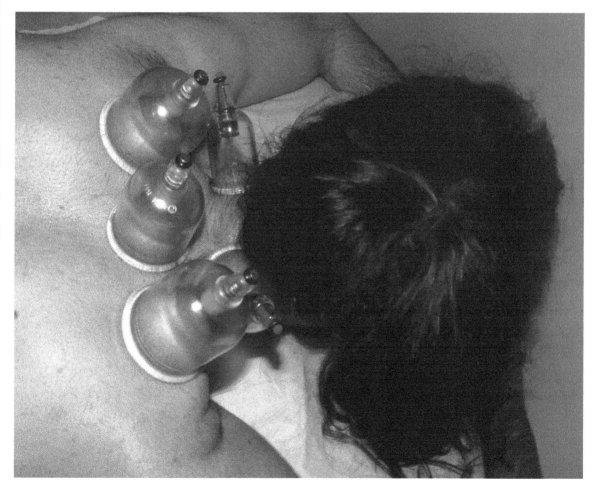

Figure 7.9: Choose small-size cups when treating neck injuries

Discus

ANATOMY INVOLVED

The discus throw dates to the ancient Olympics and is depicted in Myron's classic statue *Discobolus* as a symbol of power and strength. Today's modern track and field athlete continues the quest to throw the discus as far as possible. Success in the event requires the ability to generate power from all of the major muscle groups. Throwing the discus specifically requires muscles to exert the most amount of force in the shortest amount of time, thus engaging the fast-twitch fibres.[12]

MAIN MUSCLE GROUPS USED IN THROWING A DISCUS

- Upper body: trapezius and erector spinae muscles.

- Shoulder and chest: the pectorals, deltoids and rotator cuff muscles.

- Forearm and wrist: the arm extensors and flexors.

- Lower body: the gluteals, thigh and leg muscles (quadriceps, tibialis anterior and the gastrocnemius).

MOST COMMON DISCUS-THROWING INJURIES

- Glenohumeral ligaments (GL).

- Rotator cuff muscle injuries.

- Labral tear of the hip (see **Figure 7.11**).

- Ankle sprains.[13]

12 Voza, L. (2017) 'Which muscles are used when throwing a discus?' www.livestrong.com/article/332308-muscles-used-throwing-discus

13 Rockwell, R. (2017) 'Discus Thrower Injuries.' https://www.livestrong.com/article/discus-thrower-injuries

Discus

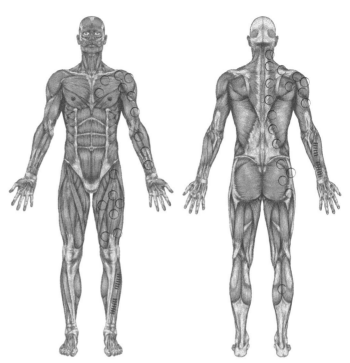

Figure 7.10: Potential discus-throwing injuries and cupping therapy locations

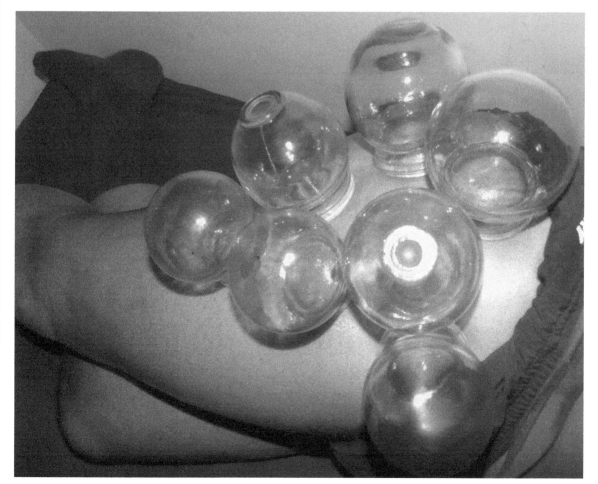

Figure 7.11: Choose large cups when treating labral tear of the hip

Football

ANATOMY INVOLVED

Football is a contact team sport with high-level risk of collision and injury.[14] During a game of football, almost all the skeletal muscles are in action. Footballers do not continuously run at the same pace. Football is an intermittent, multi-movement game in which the players are expected not only to run at different intensities, but also to tackle, pass, dribble, head and shoot. In a typical game, they perform more than 1000 changes in activity and use more than 420 different patterns of movement. The ball is in play for less than 60 minutes, with average bursts of activity lasting 4–6 seconds over distances of 14–18 metres. On average, a player will touch the ball for less than two minutes per game. Movement percentages in a game of football have been calculated as follows: walking/standing 28%, jogging 26%, running (low speed) 21%, running at moderate speed 14%, running at high speed 6%, running in sprint 3% and running backwards 2%.[15]

MAIN MUSCLE GROUPS USED IN FOOTBALL

- Upper body: deltoids, trapezius, abdominals, erector spinae, obliques and gluteals.

- Lower body: quadriceps, hamstring, gastrocnemius and soleus.

MOST COMMON FOOTBALL INJURIES

- Head and face.

- Neck, spine and back.

- Shoulder and chest.

- Wrist, hands and fingers.

- Abdomen, hip and groin.

- Upper leg.

- Knee.

- Lower leg.

- Ankle, foot, and toes[16] (see **Figure 7.13**).

14 British Medical Association (2010) *The BMA Guide to Sports Injuries.* London: Dorling Kindersley.

15 Pearson, A. (2007) *SAQ Football: Mechanics of Movement.* London: A&C Black.

16 British Medical Association (2010) *The BMA Guide to Sports Injuries.* London: Dorling Kindersley.

Football

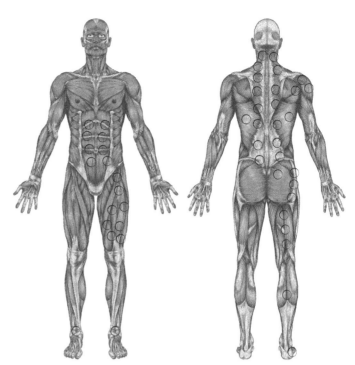

Figure 7.12: Potential football injuries and cupping therapy locations

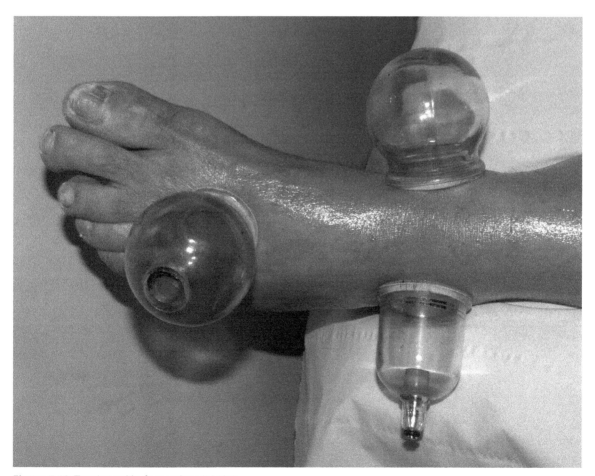

Figure 7.13: Treating ankle, foot and toe injuries

Knee, lower leg, ankle and foot injuries are the most frequently seen sporting injuries during a football match

Net-based sports (basketball, netball, volleyball)

ANATOMY INVOLVED

Net-based sports such as basketball, netball and volleyball are non-contact sport activities. They are among the most popular sports activities around the world. Athletes do not require huge muscles, but rather lean, strong and flexible muscles. All net-based sports involve running, bending, pivoting, twisting and jumping. In a game, speed, stamina and coordination are essential requirements. Strong leg muscles, particularly quadriceps, hamstrings and calf muscles, are an advantage.

MAIN MUSCLE GROUPS USED IN NET-BASED SPORTS

- Upper body: latissimus dorsi, deltoids, pectorals, rotator cuff, triceps brachii and biceps brachii.

- Lower body: hip and leg muscles – gluteals, hamstring, quadriceps and gastrocnemius.

MOST COMMON NET-BASED SPORTS INJURIES

- Neck, spine and back (see **Figure 7.15**).

- Shoulder and chest.

- Arm and elbow.

- Wrist, hand and fingers (see **Figure 7.17**).

- Abdomen, hip and groin.

- Upper leg.

- Knee.

- Lower leg.

- Ankle, foot and toes.[17]

17   British Medical Association (2010) *The BMA Guide to Sports Injuries*. London: Dorling Kindersley.

Net-based sports
(basketball, netball, volleyball)

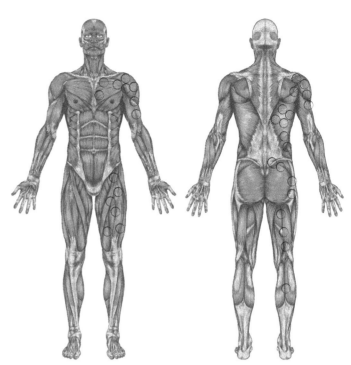

Figure 7.14: Potential net-based sports injuries and cupping therapy locations

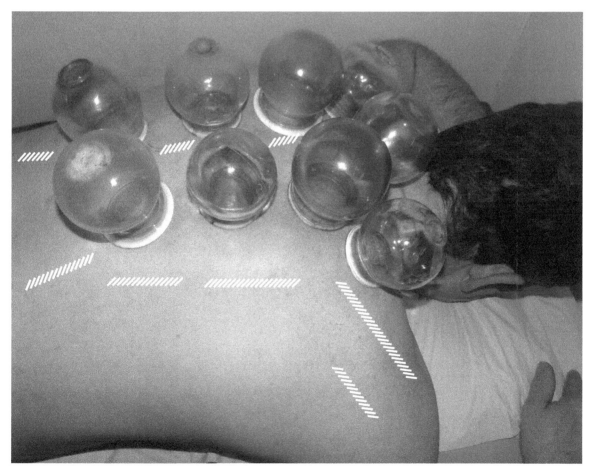

Figure 7.15: When treating neck, spine or back injuries, in addition to static cupping, I would also recommend sliding cupping application. This action will help stagnant blood to disperse, helping the muscle to recover more quickly.

Racket-based sports (badminton, squash, table tennis, tennis)

ANATOMY INVOLVED

Most racket-based sports (ball over net) such as badminton, squash, table tennis and tennis are fast-paced sports activities that require extensive use of both upper and lower body anatomy. Cardiovascular stamina is required for competitive play, which places considerable demands on the musculoskeletal system, most particularly the legs, knees, ankles, midsection, upper body and arms.

MAIN MUSCLE GROUPS USED IN RACKET-BASED SPORTS

- Leg muscles: particularly the quadriceps, hamstring and gluteus muscles as well as gastrocnemius and soleus muscles of the lower leg.

- Chest and upper-body muscles: the pectoralis major, latissimus dorsi and deltoid muscles of the torso.

- Shoulder and arm muscles: the rotator cuff, shoulder adductor and biceps and triceps muscles of the racket arm.

- Muscles of the wrist and hand.

- Lower back muscles, particularly the spinal erectors.

- Abdominal muscles: rectus abdominis, right internal and left external obliques.

- Neck muscles, in particular the neck flexor and extensor muscles.

Strength training and flexibility exercises targeting all of the above areas are essential for competitive players.[18]

MOST COMMON RACKET-BASED SPORTS INJURIES

- Neck, spine and back.
- Shoulder and chest.
- Arm and elbow.
- Wrist, hand and fingers (see **Figure 7.17**).

- Abdomen, hip and groin.
- Knee.
- Lower leg.
- Ankle, foot and toes.[19]

18   Walker, B. (2017) 'Tennis stretches and flexibility exercises', StretchCoach website, http://stretchcoach. com/articles/stretches-for-tennis

19   British Medical Association (2010) *The BMA Guide to Sports Injuries.* London: Dorling Kindersley.

Racket-based sports (badminton, squash, table tennis, tennis)

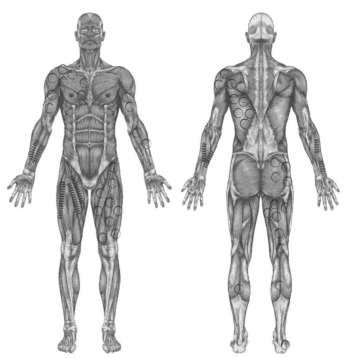

Figure 7.16: Potential racket-based sports injuries and cupping therapy locations

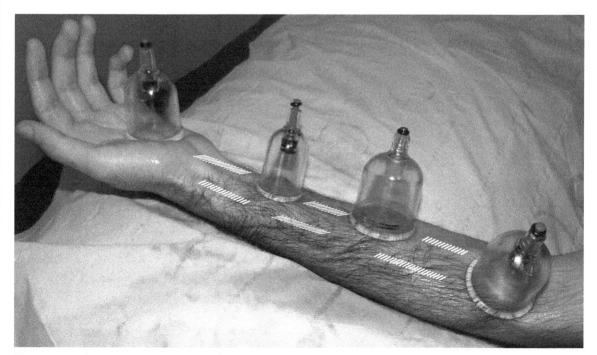

Figure 7.17: When treating wrist, hand and finger injuries, additional application of the sliding cupping technique is also recommended

Running

ANATOMY INVOLVED

Are we born to run? My answer to this age-old question is yes and no! Yes, when we are faced with a 'fight-or-flight' situation. Of course, early humans also did a lot of running for their food! And no, for running 26-mile marathons, unless you are Haile Gebrselassie, Paula Radcliffe or Sir Mo Farah!

As a child, growing up in a village, I don't remember walking much! As youngsters up to the age of 12 years old, we always ran! When I was sent out of the house for an errand and was late returning, my mother would always ask, 'What kept you so long?' or say, 'You didn't run fast enough!' After the age of 12, somehow we all began to run less and walked or cycled more. Today, however, many competitive sports activities entail some degree of running. Some may include gentle runs but many require athletes to be very fast.

> Running due to its repetitive nature places an enormous stress on human musculoskeletal system, particularly the bones, joints, tendons and other soft tissue structures that reside south of the pelvis. If we plan our running sessions well and allow recovery, then these tissues adapt and the body does not find itself in a state of perpetual breakdown. If, however, we do not allow adequate recovery (a very individual time frame) then the runner will suffer some manner of running-affected injury.[20]

The strain placed on the lower limbs means that short-, middle- and long-distance runners all suffer injury.

MAIN MUSCLE GROUPS USED IN RUNNING

- Upper body: abdominals, hip flexors (iliopsoas), gluteals.

- Lower body: hamstrings, quadriceps, tibialis anterior, gastrocnemius and the proneal muscles.

MOST COMMON RUNNING INJURIES

- Neck.
- Spine.
- Back.
- Abdomen.
- Hip.

- Groin.
- Upper leg (see **Figure 7.19**).
- Knee.
- Lower leg.
- Ankle, foot and toes.[21]

....

20   Mallac, C., The Sports Injury Doctor website, www.sportsinjurybulletin.com, Bulletin No. 126.

21   British Medical Association (2010) *The BMA Guide to Sports Injuries.* London: Dorling Kindersley.

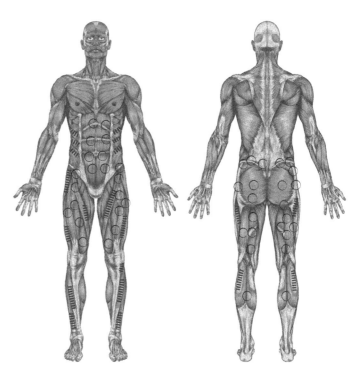

Figure 7.18: Potential running injuries and cupping therapy locations

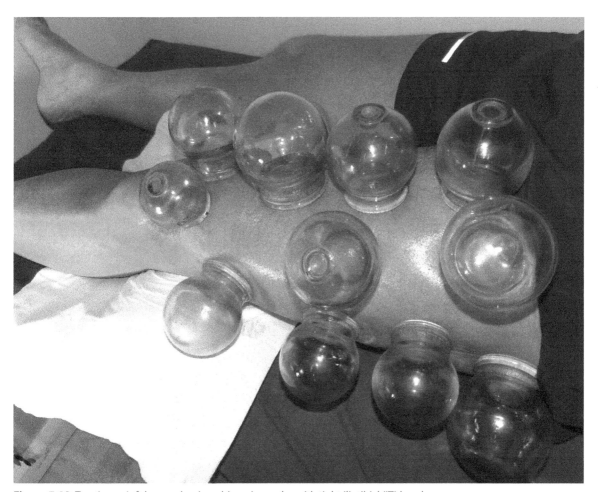

Figure 7.19: Treating painful upper-leg (quadriceps) muscles with tight iliotibial (IT) band

Ski-based sports (skiing, waterskiing)

ANATOMY INVOLVED

Ski-based sports are considered to be high-risk activities. These sports put tremendous strain on the knees, ankles and hips, and therefore require good stability in the lower limbs.[22]

MAIN MUSCLE GROUPS USED IN SKI-BASED SPORTS

- Upper body: the core muscles and deltoids.

- Lower body: gluteal muscles, quadriceps, hamstrings, biceps femoris and knee flexors and extensors.

MOST COMMON SKI-BASED SPORTS INJURIES

- Head and face.

- Neck, spine and back.

- Shoulder and chest.

- Elbow and arm.

- Wrist, hand and fingers.

- Abdomen, hip and groin (see **Figure 7.21**).

- Upper leg.

- Knee.

- Ankle, foot and toes.[23]

22   British Medical Association (2010) *The BMA Guide to Sports Injuries*. London: Dorling Kindersley.

23   British Medical Association (2010) *The BMA Guide to Sports Injuries*. London: Dorling Kindersley.

Ski-based sports
(skiing, waterskiing)

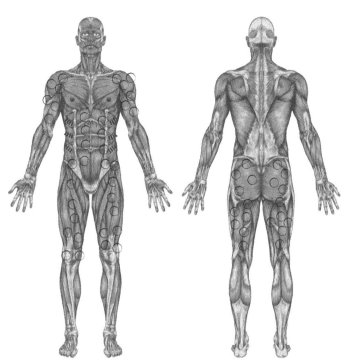

Figure 7.20: Potential ski-based sports injuries and cupping therapy locations

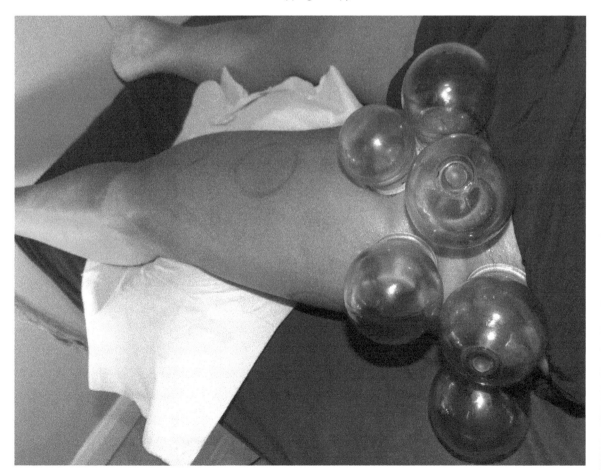

Figure 7.21: Employ light to medium-strength suction when treating the groin and abdominal areas, and stronger suction when working on the hip joint

Swimming

ANATOMY INVOLVED

Swimming is truly a full-body workout activity, where the entire musculoskeletal system is activated. Swimming is considered to be a low-risk sport. Nevertheless, swimming puts a great deal of stress on the muscles, particularly the back and shoulders.

MAIN MUSCLE GROUPS USED IN SWIMMING

In all four types of swimming techniques (breaststroke, backstroke, front crawl and butterfly):

- Upper body: the core muscles, deltoids, biceps, triceps, trapezius, pectorals, latissimus dorsi, rectus abdominis and external obliques.

- Lower body: gluteals, quadriceps, hamstrings, gastrocnemius, tibialis anterior, the feet (abductor hallucius and flexor digitorium brevis).

MOST COMMON SWIMMING INJURIES

- Hand and face.

- Neck, spine and back.

- Shoulder and chest (see **Figure 7.23**).

- Arm and elbow.

- Wrist, hand and fingers.

- Abdomen, hip and groin.

- Knee.[24]

....

24   British Medical Association (2010) *The BMA Guide to Sports Injuries.* London: Dorling Kindersley.

....

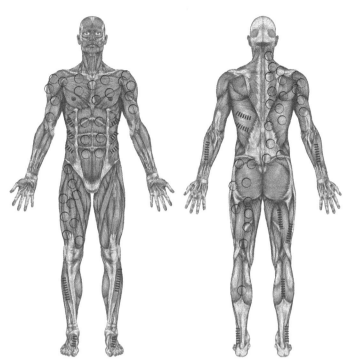

Figure 7.22: Potential swimming injuries and cupping therapy locations

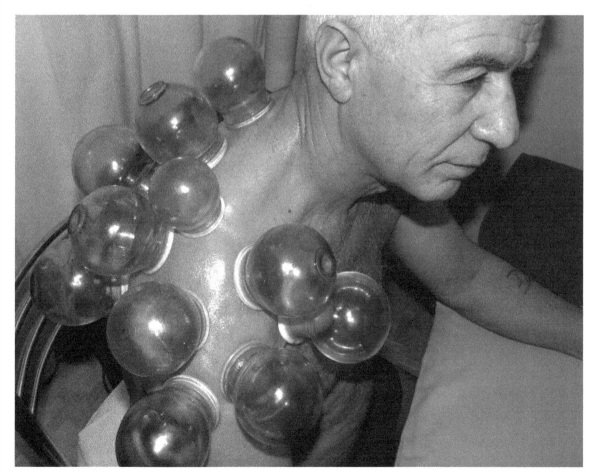

Figure 7.23: Apply medium-strength suction when treating the chest muscles, and stronger suction when treating shoulder muscle injuries

Water sports (rowing, kayaking, canoeing, sailing, white water rafting, sculling)

ANATOMY INVOLVED

Water sports such as kayaking, rowing and canoeing put strain on the shoulders, forearms and wrists due to repeated arm movements.[25] Back pain is also a common complaint.

MAIN MUSCLE GROUPS USED IN WATER SPORTS

- Upper body: deltoids, trapezius, erector spinae, rhomboids, pectoralis major, rectus abdominis, triceps and wrist extensors.

- Lower body: quadriceps, hamstrings, gastrocnemius, soleus muscles.

MOST COMMON WATER SPORTS INJURIES

- Neck, spine and back.

- Shoulder and chest.

- Arm and elbow.

- Wrist, hands and fingers.

- Abdomen, hips and groin.

- Knee.

- Ankle, foot and toes.[26]

....

25   British Medical Association (2010) *The BMA Guide to Sports Injuries*. London: Dorling Kindersley.

26   British Medical Association (2010) *The BMA Guide to Sports Injuries*. London: Dorling Kindersley.

....

Water sports
(rowing, kayaking,
canoeing, sailing, white
water rafting, sculling)

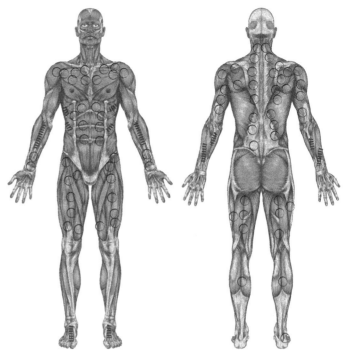

Figure 7.24: Potential water sports injuries
and cupping therapy locations

Weightlifting and powerlifting

ANATOMY INVOLVED

Any activity that involves heavy lifting puts enormous pressure and stress on the entire musculoskeletal system, particularly on the ligaments, tendons and joints.

MAIN MUSCLE GROUPS USED IN WEIGHTLIFTING AND POWERLIFTING

- Shoulder muscles: trapezius, deltoids.

- Chest muscles: pectorals (major and minor).

- Upper arms: triceps and biceps.

- Wrist: flexors and extensors.

- Abdominals: rectus abdominis and obliques.

- Back: latissimus dorsi, rhomboids and erector spinae.

- Hips: gluteals.

- Thighs: quadriceps and hamstrings.

- Calves: gastrocnemius and soleus muscles.[27]

MOST COMMON WEIGHTLIFTING AND POWERLIFTING INJURIES

- Neck, spine and back (see **Figures 7.25 and 7.26**).

- Shoulder and chest.

- Arm and elbow.

- Abdomen, hip and groin.

- Knee.[28]

....

27   British Medical Association (2010) *The BMA Guide to Sports Injuries*. London: Dorling Kindersley.

28   British Medical Association (2010) *The BMA Guide to Sports Injuries*. London: Dorling Kindersley.

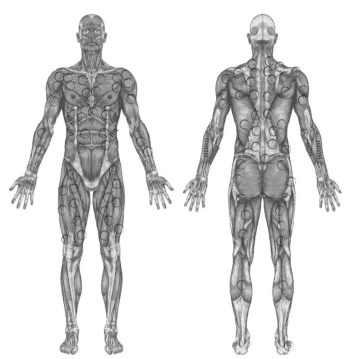

Figure 7.25: Potential weightlifting and powerlifting injuries and cupping therapy locations

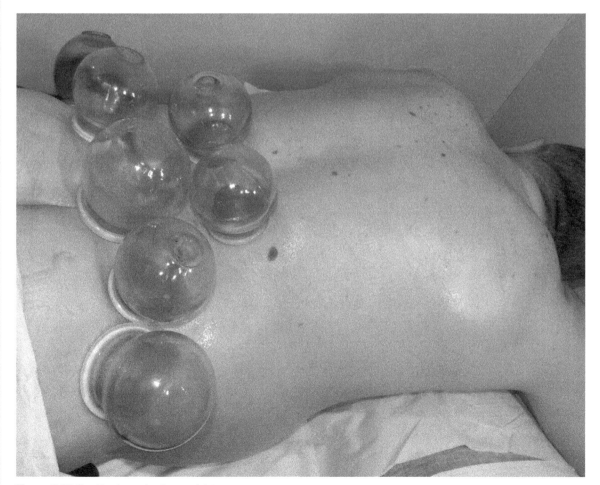

Figure 7.26: Treating lower back complaints

.... ◆ ◆ ◆ ....

CHAPTER 8

COSMETIC CUPPING THERAPY

Why is cupping massage so unique?

The answer to this question is concealed within the innermost layer of the skin, namely the dermis … and I like to call it 'TCT Factor' (The Connective Tissue Factor).

By the nature of the cupping application, an unavoidable and intimate association is established between cupping and the dermis. The dermis, the innermost layer of the skin, is composed of about 80% connective tissue called collagen and elastin. It also contains blood and lymph vessels, sweat glands which regulate body temperature, hair follicles, sebaceous glands that produce sebum (an oily substance which lubricates and keeps the skin moist) and an intricate network of sensory nerves. Collagen and elastin are protein fibres which support our structure and hold body parts together – the true building blocks of our body. Both of these wonderful structural proteins are the most fundamental skin fibres which provide our skin with necessary firmness and elasticity. Collagen gives our skin firmness and strength while elastin provides elasticity and expansion (reduced skin elasticity causes wrinkles to appear). Elastin is also present in artery walls, bones, cartilage, ligaments, the lungs and intestines, helping them to stretch and expand and return to their original form. In the event of skin tissue damage (a cut or wound), dermal fibroblast cells are stimulated in order to produce wound-healing proteins, namely collagen and elastin.

I believe that, at this juncture, the physical link between cause and effect of the cupping application becomes obvious. As cupping massage mimics an external physical attack on the skin surface, similar to an injury, the fibroblast cells are tricked into repair mode, thus increasing production of collagen and elastin, the wound-healing proteins which help to repair the skin tissue, giving the skin's surface fuller, softer lines with a fresher, healthier, youthful look.

However, as we get older – that is, past 30! –our natural collagen and elastin production slows down. Our body will continue to produce both proteins throughout our life but at a much reduced rate. As collagen and elastin production is reduced, the skin becomes less resilient to the forces of nature – namely, gravity! Connective tissue damage also occurs as a result of long-term exposures to the sun's UV radiation, as well as excessive use of chemical skin peelers. As far as I am aware, there is not a single product available that will reverse this process entirely.

Expensive collagen and elastin creams, chemical skin peelers and laser treatments are frequently advertised by the cosmetic industry. I believe that cupping massage stimulation is the most natural and effective way to boost and maintain connective tissue regeneration. This is why. When massaging the skin with bare hands, the therapist decides which type of massage technique to use. Stroking, rolling, pinching, kneading, pressure, percussion or pulling methods are mostly employed. With cupping massage, however, all the above movements are combined in one action. Consequently, when a cup is applied statically or moved along the skin, the negative pressure inside the cup causes decompression and deep tissue manipulation to the local myofascia; it creates friction, pulls, pinches, rolls and kneads, all at the same time! Only the intensity of the suction will vary. Through cupping application, dead skin is peeled off (exfoliation) and lymph glands are activated, boosting the immune system and helping to clear waste away (detoxification).

Meanwhile, oxygen-rich blood is channelled into the micro-blood vessels (oxygen saturation), nourishing the entire connective tissue, resulting in healthier, fuller and younger-looking skin (rejuvenation).

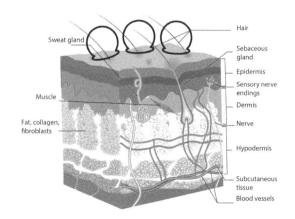

Figure 8.1: Skin and fascia in relation to cupping therapy application

Before you start

No matter what type of massage you are about to employ, there are few basic rules that must be observed. One of the most important details is the comfort of the treatment room. It must be warm with a comfortable massage mat or table. Next is the type of massage oil to be used. Confirm with your patient that they are not allergic to the oil you are about to use. If they are not sure, apply a few drops of the massage oil to the patient's skin and wait for 30 minutes to see if any reaction develops. My favoured massage oils are almond oil, coconut oil and olive oil.

A WORD OF CAUTION

Avoid over-treatment, particularly during the first and second visits. Gently introduce cupping massage to your patients by keeping the suction light as well as limiting the cupping movements to not more than five movements during the initial two visits. Cupping movements can be increased by increments of five on follow-up treatments, up to a maximum of 50 movements on each location.

Cosmetic cupping techniques

Facial cupping massage (the natural way to facial rejuvenation)

The face is considered to be the 'mirror' of a person's health. To the outside world, both the physical and the emotional state of affairs are expressed through our face. This is because the face contains a massive number of nerve receptors which are intimately linked with the central nervous system. I'm sure that at some point in our lives we have all been able to observe happiness, contentment and joy as well as pain, anger, restlessness and frustration just by looking at a friend's face, and have asked, 'Is everything all right?'

In my clinic, facial cupping massage is one of the most frequently requested treatments.

- Cupping massage to the face softens facial lines, brings colour and energy, helps disperse anxiety and the 'tired look', benefiting complexion and appearance.

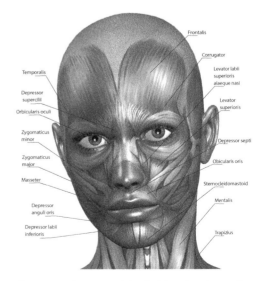

Figure 8.2: Anatomy of the facial and neck muscles

Anatomy of the facial and neck muscles

In order to get the best results from facial cupping massage, it is necessary to know the muscular make-up of the face and the neck. The cupping massage technique you are about to employ will very much depend on knowing the position and the function of the muscle group you are working on. For the treatment to be most effective, the movement of the cup should follow the curve and contour of the muscle and not cross it.

The facial muscles are a set of about 20 smooth skeletal muscles lying under the facial skin. Most of them originate from the skull or fibrous structures and radiate to the skin through an elastic tendon. The facial muscles are positioned around the facial openings (mouth, eye, nose and ear) or stretch across the skull and neck.

Preparing for facial cupping massage

Recommended cupping equipment

- Rubber-top cupping set (**Figure 8.3**).

- Silicon cups (**Figure 8.4**).

- Pistol-handled cupping set (**Figure 8.5**).

> **A WORD OF CAUTION**
> Avoid using the fire cupping technique on the face.

Treatment position

It is best to have the patient in a supine position (lying face upwards). The practitioner sits or stands behind the patient, gaining full access to the head, face and neck (**Figure 8.6A, B**). I recommend using both hands during the cupping massage – one hand to hold the cup firmly and the free hand to support the skin while the cup is moved.

Step 1: With bare hands, massage and warm the entire face, including the forehead, ears, chin, under the chin and the neck, with massage oil of your choice. This also helps to establish rapport with your patient at the start of the session.

Step 2: Once the face massage is completed, choose a small suction cup which will be suitable to work on the facial muscles. Facial cupping massage consists of 11 cupping movements (CM).

Facial cupping massage protocol

Third eye

CM 1: Start the facial cupping massage from the midpoint between the eyebrows (this point is also referred as the 'spiritual point' or the 'third-eye chakra'). Engage the cup on the third eye. While using one hand to move the cup on the skin, use your free hand to

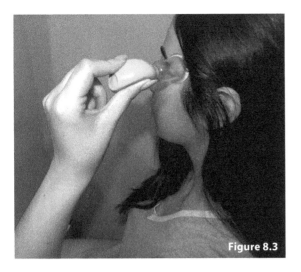

Figure 8.3

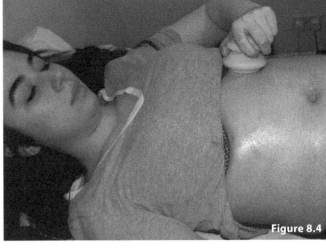

Figure 8.4

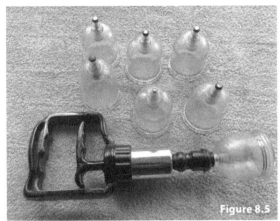

Figure 8.5

Figure 8.3: Cupping massage using rubber/silicon-top cupping set

Figure 8.4: Self-cupping massage with silicon cups

Figure 8.5: Pistol-handled cupping set

Figure 8.6A, B: Practitioner positioning himself behind the patient

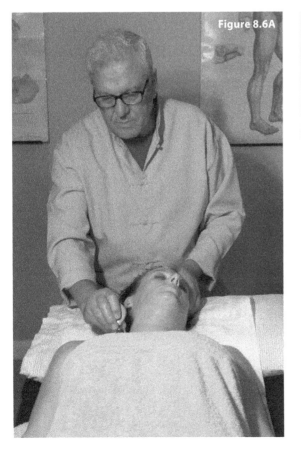

Figure 8.6A

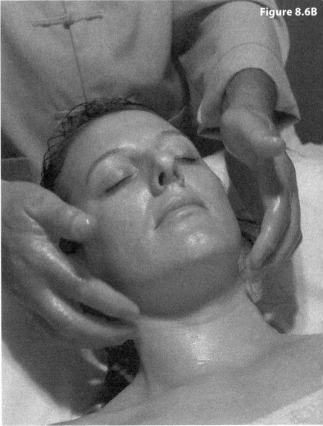

Figure 8.6B

support the skin behind the moving cup. Slide the cup towards the hairline. Remove the suction cup and repeat the cupping massage from the point at which you started. Repeat the same movement no more than five times during the first and second visits. This can be increased by five movements each following week to a maximum of 50 movements on each muscle group in one given session. This is a gentle way to introduce cupping stimulation to the facial muscle groups. While massaging, always monitor the skin's reaction and modify your technique accordingly. If the colour of the skin goes beyond pinkish-red to bright red or, worse, to dark red, stop the treatment immediately, reduce the strength of suction and try again. Should you lose the suction as you move the cup (which happens often), reapply and continue with the treatment. Avoid applying pressure on the cup while moving it on the skin surface. The movement should be smooth and effortless. Should the patient complain of pain or discomfort while you are moving the cup, this could be a sign of strong suction or dry skin, which can be remedied by applying weaker suction or additional massage oil.

• Cupping massage to the 'third-eye chakra' is believed to stimulate the pineal gland located deep in the centre of the brain, responsible for the endocrine system which produces the hormone melatonin. Melatonin helps to maintain the circadian rhythm (24-hour biological clock), regulate the reproductive system in men and women, and relax the mind and clear the head (**Figure 8.7A, B**).

Forehead

CM 2: Starting from just above the eyebrows, apply and move the cup upwards, towards the hairline (**Figure 8.8A**).

CM 3: Starting from the middle of the forehead, slide the cup laterally towards the temple (**Figure 8.8B**).

Because of the fine skin at the forehead, it is quite common to lose suction frequently while moving the cup at this location. In this case, persevere, removing and reapplying the cup, and continue with the treatment.

• Cupping massage to the forehead helps to reduce lines and gets rid of tension headaches.

Under the eyes

CM 4: Massage under the eyes, starting from the base of the nose and moving laterally towards the temple. Repeat the movement five times. Extra care is necessary when cupping under the eyes, since the skin under the eyes is the thinnest on the human body. Repeat to the opposite side (**Figure 8.9A, B, C**).

- Cupping massage around the eyes relaxes tired eyes and brings energy to the eye muscle and the optic nerve.

- It also helps to relieve nasal congestion.

Lips

CM 5: Upper lip. Choose a small cup to administer lip massage. The movement is from one corner of the mouth to the other. Continue with cupping massage from the corner of the mouth towards the temple, then towards the eyes and finally towards the inner canthus of the eyes (**Figure 8.10**).

CM 6: The lower-lip massage is a similar movement to the upper-lip massage. Continue with the lower-lip massage from the corner of the mouth laterally, aiming towards the ear lobe (**Figure 8.11**).

- Cupping massage around the lips helps to reduce wrinkles around the mouth.

Face

CM 7: Side of the face. Following the jawline, start the cupping massage from the lower jaw and move the cup towards the ear and the outer corner of the eye. Repeat the same action to the opposite side of the face (**Figure 8.12A, B, C**).

- This technique softens facial lines, brings energy and colour to the cheeks and helps reduce facial tension.

Chin

CM 8: Massage the chin by moving and sliding the cup from side to side over the chin bone (mandible).

NB. Extra care is needed when massaging the chin, as this area is known to bruise quite easily.

Under the chin

CM 9: Start the cupping massage from the tip of the chin and move the cup in a medial direction towards the throat, reaching to the top of the sternum. Next, move the cup from the throat cartilage laterally (outwards) towards the neck. Repeat the same movements to the opposite side (**Figure 8.14A, B, C**).

• Cupping massage application under the chin tightens the local muscles and prevents sagging (double chin).

Neck

CM 10: Neck muscle (sternocleidomastoid). Starting from under the ear, massage and move the cup towards the collarbone (clavicle). With neck muscles, cupping massage can be applied in both directions – that is, from the collarbone upwards towards the ear and vice versa. Repeat the massage to the opposite side (**Figure 8.15A, B, C**).

• Cupping massage to the neck helps reduce tension and anxiety, and improves blood circulation to the head.

• Massaging the neck muscle tightens and restores skin elasticity and reduces wrinkles.

Upper chest

CM 11: Under the collarbone and top of the chest. Starting from the middle of the chest (sternum), move the cup under the collarbone laterally (outwards), over the chest muscle (pectoralis major) towards the tip of the shoulder. Repeat the movement to the opposite side (**Figure 8.16A, B, C**).

• Massaging under the collarbone and the upper chest tightens the chest muscle and reduces wrinkles.

> **A WORD OF CAUTION**
> Avoid cupping massage on the collarbone if there is a recent history of injury or fracture. Avoid strong cupping on the face, neck and chest.

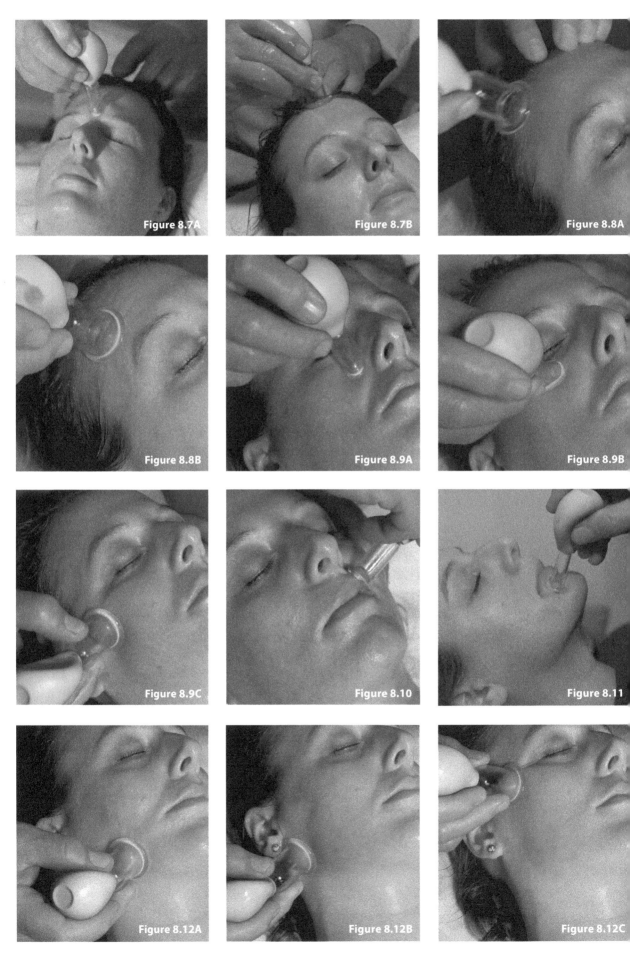

Figure 8.7A

Figure 8.7B

Figure 8.8A

Figure 8.8B

Figure 8.9A

Figure 8.9B

Figure 8.9C

Figure 8.10

Figure 8.11

Figure 8.12A

Figure 8.12B

Figure 8.12C

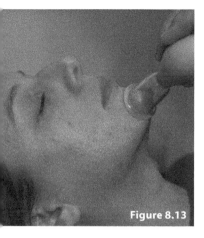

Figure 8.13

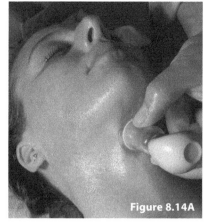

Figure 8.14A

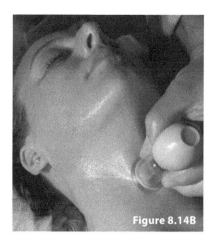

Figure 8.14B

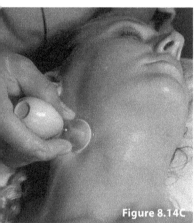

Figure 8.14C

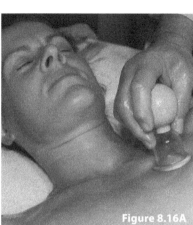

Figure 8.16A

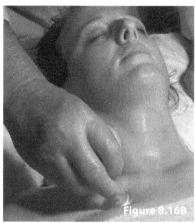

Figure 8.16B

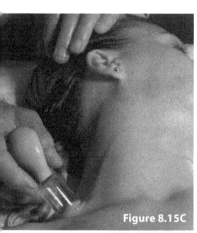

Figure 8.15C

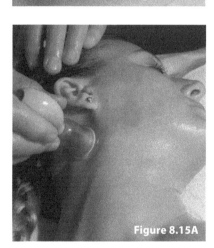

Figure 8.15A

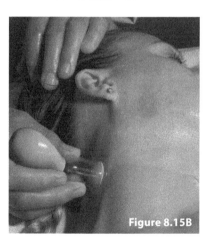

Figure 8.15B

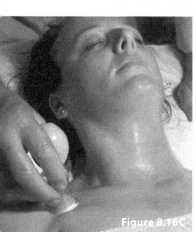

Figure 8.16C

Facing page:

Figure 8.7A, B: Begin the treatment from the third-eye chakra

Figure 8.8A, B: Forehead
A. Move the cup towards the hairline, starting from just above the eyebrow; B. Move the cup across the forehead

Figure 8.9A, B, C: Cupping massage under the eyes
Start the treatment from the corner of the nose and move the cup laterally, towards the outer corner of the eye

Figure 8.10: Upper lip
Choose a small-size cup and move from side to side, following the contour of the lip muscle

Figure 8.11: Lower lip
Massage from one corner of the mouth to the opposite corner

Figure 8.12A, B, C: Facial cupping massage (side of the face)

This page:

Figure 8.13: Chin

Figure 8.14A, B, C: Under the chin

Figure 8.15A, B, C: Neck muscle (sternocleidomastoid)

Figure 8.16A, B, C: Under the collarbone and top of the chest

Cupping massage protocol for shoulders, arms and hands

Continue with the cupping massage treatment to the shoulders, arms and hands, without altering the patient's position.

Shoulder, arm and hand cupping massage consists of six cupping movements (CM).

Shoulder

CM 1: Using a medium-size single cup (glass or silicon), begin the cupping massage from the tip of the shoulder (head of the humerus and deltoid muscle). In order to massage the whole of the deltoid muscle, apply light to medium-strength cupping and rotate and move the cup following the contour of the deltoid muscle (**Figure 8.17**).

Upper arms

CM 2: Upper arms (triceps brachii and biceps brachii), front of the arms. From the tip of the shoulder (deltoid muscle), work towards the elbow. Use long cupping strokes rather than short, sharp strokes. Each time lift the cup from the elbow and return to the head of the shoulder to repeat the same action (**Figure 8.18A, B**).

Back of the arms

CM 3: Upper arms, back muscle (brachialis and triceps). When applying cupping massage to the back of the arms, use light suction, as these areas are quite tender parts of the arm. In order to facilitate lymphatic drainage, finish off the treatment by massaging from the inside of the elbow, working up towards the underarm (**Figure 8.19**).

Lower arms

CM 4: Outer forearms (extensor muscles). Start cupping massage from the elbow, move the cup towards the back of the wrist and return to the elbow position (**Figure 8.20A, B**). Always replenish the massage oil on the skin when moving the cup becomes harder.

Forearms

CM 5: Inside of the forearms (and flexor muscles). Apply light cupping to the inside of the elbow and move the cup towards the front of the wrist. Finish by returning to the inner elbow position (**Figure 8.21A, B**). Continue cupping massage from the inside of the elbow and finish off at the armpit.

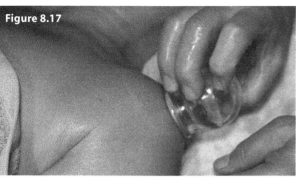

Figure 8.17

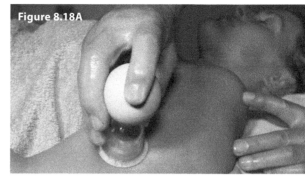

Figure 8.18A

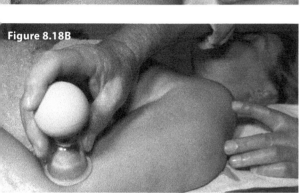

Figure 8.18B

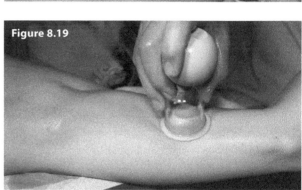

Figure 8.19

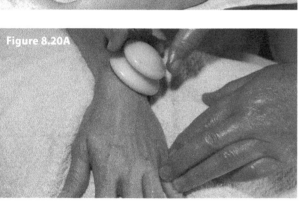

Figure 8.20A

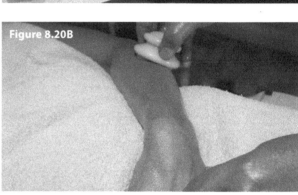

Figure 8.20B

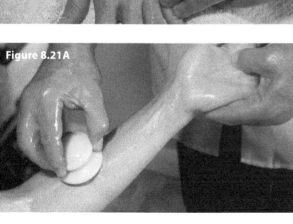

Figure 8.21A

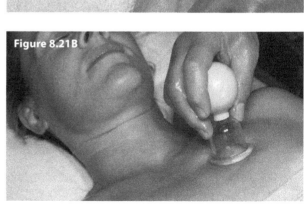

Figure 8.21B

Figure 8.22

Figure 8.17: Shoulder

Figure 8.18A, B: Upper arms (triceps brachii and biceps brachii)

Figure 8.19: Back of the arms (brachialis and triceps)

Figure 8.20A, B: Outer forearms (extensor muscles)

Figure 8.21A, B: Forearms

Figure 8.22: Cupping the palm

Palm

CM 6: Apply medium-strength to strong cupping inside the palm, using two small cups or one large cup, and leave in position for several minutes. Finish off the treatment by pulling and twisting each finger (**Figure 8.22**).

Cupping massage to the arms and hands:

- encourages blood circulation
- relaxes muscle, ligaments and tendons
- brings energy to the extremities
- promotes lymphatic circulation.

Cupping massage protocol for chest and breast

Chest

CM 1: Using light to medium-strength suction, start the chest cupping massage from the middle of the chest (sternum/breastbone). Move and slide the cup laterally (outwards) on and over the chest muscle (pectoralis major) towards the shoulder, sliding the cup in a half-moon motion. Repeat the same procedure to the opposite side of the chest (**Figure 8.23A, B, C**).

Under the breast

CM 2: Start the cupping massage from the tip of the sternum (xiphoid process of the sternum), sliding and moving the cup laterally towards the armpit. Disengage the cup and repeat the procedure, making sure that you slide the cup laterally, starting from the middle of the chest and moving outwards (**Figure 8.24A, B**).

- Cupping massage to the chest helps to relax the muscles between the ribcage, opens up the chest and benefits breathing.

Breast

CM 1: Apply massage oil liberally to the entire breast. Choose a small cup, making sure that the edges are soft and smooth. Obtain a light suction and commence cupping from the base of the breast (on the pectoralis major muscle), moving the cup clockwise around the outside of the breast, circling and massaging the whole breast. Five cupping movements, increasing to 30–50 in the coming weeks, is the typical method (**Figure 8.25**).

CM 2: Cupping massage on the breast. When the circling cupping massage is completed, use a specially manufactured breast cup with a control valve, which is used to adjust the pressure inside the cup, and apply it on the breast, including the nipple, initially for five minutes, increasing to 15 minutes in follow-up visits (**Figure 8.26**).

The patient should experience no pain whatsoever during this procedure. However, if there is any sign of breast pain, remove the cup and reapply employing lighter suction. Breasts can be very tender; therefore, always begin the treatment with light cupping application and increase to medium strength in the following weeks. *Never apply strong cupping on the breast as it may cause discharge or bleeding from the nipple.*

Cupping massage to the base of the breasts:

- helps tighten and tone the tendons, preventing sagging

- stimulates the production of anti-aging hormones such as prolactin, oxytocin and oestrogen

- increases blood flow to the breast

- helps with lymphatic drainage of the breast

- stimulates the mammary glands

- increases breast size.

A WORD OF CAUTION
Refrain from breast cupping:

- if the patient is below 15 years of age

- if there is any sign of breast inflammation, swelling or lump

- if the patient experiences pain or there is any form of discharge

- if there are size abnormalities between the breasts

- if there are skin texture abnormalities on or around the breast.

Avoid using strong cupping on the chest and breast.

Cupping massage protocol for abdomen

Elevate the patient's knees by placing a pillow or towel under the knees so that the back and the front core muscles are totally relaxed (**Figure 8.27A, B**). Cupping massage over the abdominal area could be sensitive, particularly if the person is going through a stressful time in their life.

Oil the entire abdomen (upper and lower abdomen).

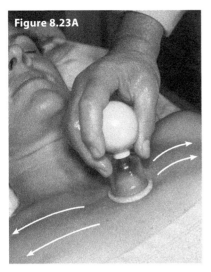
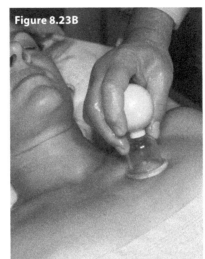
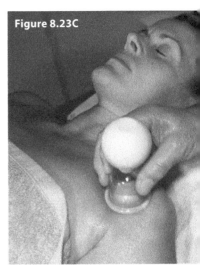

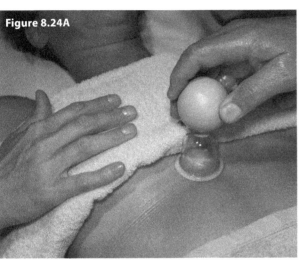
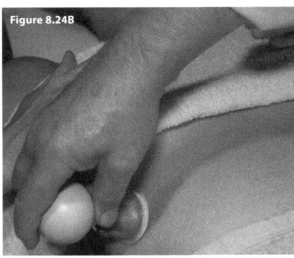

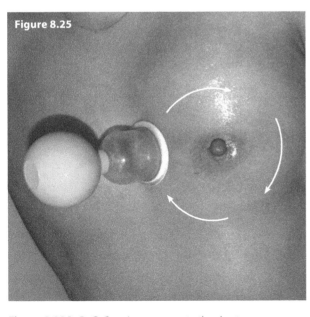
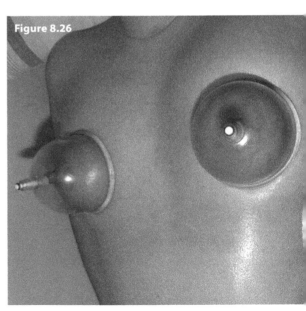

Figure 8.23A, B, C: Cupping massage to the chest
Figure 8.24A, B: Cupping massage under the breast
Figure 8.25: Cupping massage around (circling) the breast
Figure 8.26: Cupping massage on the breast

Abdomen

CM 1: Start the abdominal cupping massage by applying 10–15 light static cups over the entire abdomen for five minutes.

Diaphragm

CM 2: Draw an imaginary straight line from the tip of the sternum to the pubic bone. Using a single cup, apply light suction and move the cup on the diaphragm muscle under the ribcage. Massage the diaphragm muscle laterally towards the floating ribs. Repeat the same action from the imaginary midline, massaging the upper and the lower abdomen, finishing in line with the pubic bone (**Figure 8.28**).

Umbilical cupping massage

CM 3: After completing the lateral movement to both aspects of the abdomen, continue with cupping massage using a single cup (preferably a silicon cup) in a clockwise circular motion, starting from the umbilicus and expanding the circle as you move round the abdominal muscle (rectus abdominis) (**Figure 8.29**).

Cupping massage to abdomen:

- improves digestion
- helps with constipation and the elimination process
- firms and strengthens the abdominal core muscles
- promotes circulation of oxygen-rich blood to the internal organs
- improves blood circulation to the reproductive system (in both sexes)
- helps release tension and de-stresses in general
- soothes stomach aches and period pains
- aids the hepatic portal system, benefiting the liver and gallbladder
- improves abdominal skin texture
- helps to release muscle cramps
- softens the appearance of scar tissue
- promotes lymphatic circulation.

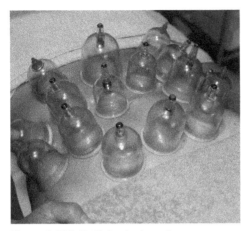
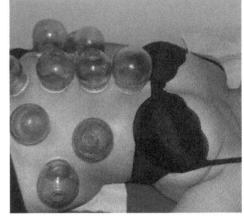

Figure 8.27A, B: Abdominal cupping

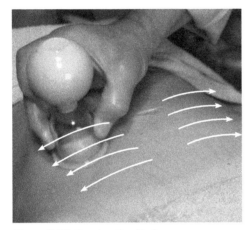
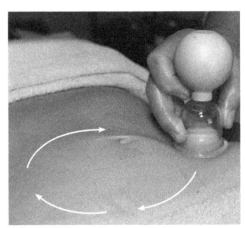

Figure 8.28: Cupping the diaphragm

Figure 8.29: Umbilical cupping massage
Move the cup clockwise in a circular motion, starting from the umbilical region and expanding outwards to the pubic bone

A WORD OF CAUTION

Avoid strong cupping application to the upper and the lower abdomen.

Cupping massage protocol for the legs (anti-cellulite massage)

Cupping massage to legs is one of the most frequently requested treatments – both for numerous cellulite-related complaints and for sports-related injuries. From my personal clinical experience of using cupping massage to treat cellulite complaints, I have found it to be the most effective method of all massage techniques. Usually, after the fifth or sixth treatment cellulite appears to become softer and smoother.

Front aspect of the legs/thighs

Have the patient in the supine position and oil the whole of the leg liberally, starting from the ankle and moving towards the top of the thigh and into the groin.

CM 1: Using glass or pistol-handled Perspex cups, apply 10–15 light-suction static cups for five minutes, cupping the entire upper leg and thigh, including the inner and outer thigh and the knee (**Figure 8.30**).

CM 2: Remove all cups after five minutes (**Figure 8.31**).

Legs

CM 3: Apply more massage oil if necessary. Choose a medium-size silicon cup, and commence the treatment by applying sliding cupping massage starting from the groin and working from the inside of the leg laterally towards the outer aspect of the thigh, altering the sliding cup position with each massage cupping movement and working the cup closer towards the knee (this stimulates the adductor muscles). When treatment of the thigh is completed, move the treatment to the frontal muscle (quadriceps femoris) and finally to the outer thigh (iliotibial tract or the IT band). Complete the treatment by applying sliding cupping to the whole upper leg, starting from the knee and moving the cup towards the groin and the lymph glands (**Figure 8.32A, B, C, D, E, F**).

Below the knee

CM 4: Using a single silicon cup, massage the lower part of the outer leg, starting from the kneecap (patella) and working towards the ankle (the flexor muscles of ankle and foot are stimulated). Repeat the same action to the inner aspect of the lower leg (**Figure 8.33A, B**).

Most leg muscle structures are long muscles; during cupping massage treatment, therefore, long strokes are more effective than short bursts.

Cupping massage to legs:

- promotes blood and fluid circulation
- is by far the most effective anti-cellulite massage technique
- helps with lymphatic drainage
- relaxes tired muscles, tendons and ligaments
- benefits stiff joints
- prevents cramps
- brings energy to the lower extremities.

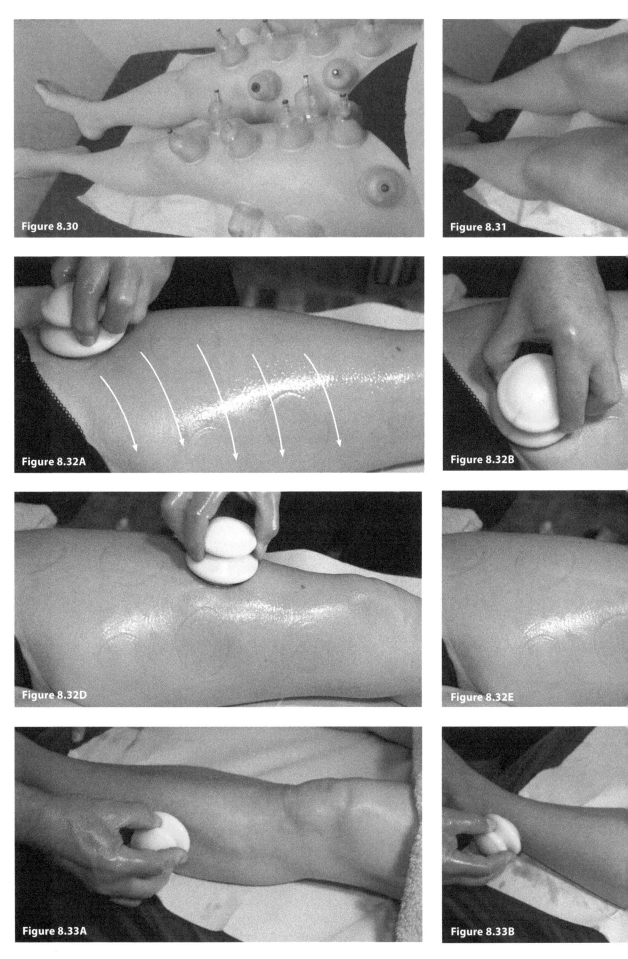

Figure 8.30

Figure 8.31

Figure 8.32A

Figure 8.32B

Figure 8.32D

Figure 8.32E

Figure 8.33A

Figure 8.33B

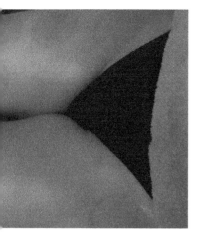

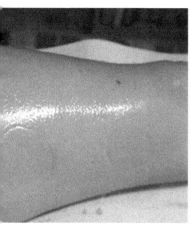

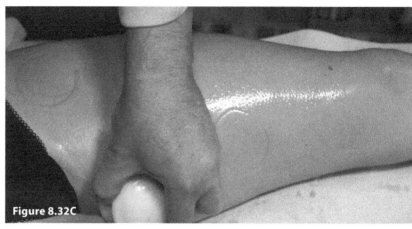

Figure 8.32C

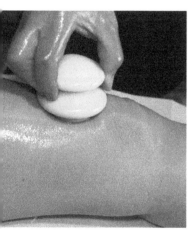

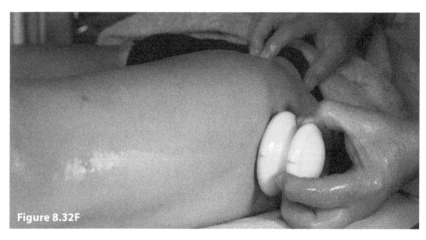

Figure 8.32F

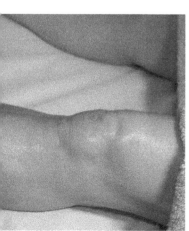

Figure 8.30: Front aspect of the legs/thighs
Figure 8.31: Remove all cups from the legs
Figure 8.32A, B, C, D, E, F: Cupping massage to the legs
Figure 8.33A, B: Below the knee

Cupping massage protocol for the back of the neck, shoulders and upper back (posterior aspect of trunk)

Place the patient in a prone (face down) position, preferably on a treatment couch with a facial opening in order to rest the patient's face comfortably. Sometimes, lying face down on a flat surface and turning the neck sideways for a long duration can be an uncomfortable experience; it can also cause neck spasm and pain.

Back of the neck

CM 1: Starting with the back of the neck, apply 2–4 small static cups with medium-strength suction for five minutes on the neck muscles, avoiding the hairline (**Figure 8.34**).

Upper back

CM 2: Continue the cupping application with larger cups, employing medium-strength suction (10–15 cups) from the shoulders (trapezius and deltoid muscles) and working downwards, covering the whole of the back (latissimus dorsi muscle), ending at the waistline, for five minutes (**Figure 8.35**).

CM 3: Remove all cups after five minutes and apply additional massage oil to all areas of the back (**Figure 8.36**).

Neck massage

CM 4: Choose a small silicon cup and massage the neck in an up-and-down motion, starting from the hairline (splenius capitis muscle) and working towards T1 (first thoracic vertebra) (**Figure 8.37A, B**).

Shoulders

CM 5: Using a single glass or silicon cup, apply light to medium-strength cupping massage, starting from T1 and working laterally towards the tip of the shoulder, covering the trapezius and deltoid muscles. (The trapezius is a large kite-shaped muscle, running across the top of the back of the neck, and the deltoid is the thick triangular muscle that caps the shoulder (**Figure 8.38A, B**).)

Posterior trunk

CM 6: Using a single glass or silicon cup, apply medium-strength suction and start cupping massage of the posterior trunk (back of the torso) at the top of the large erector spinae muscle (the erector spinae muscle is made up of a bunch of muscles and tendons and extends to the buttocks), working downwards towards the waistline, in an up-and-down motion. Apply the same method to the opposite side of the body (**Figure 8.39A, B, C**).

CM 7: Continue massaging the posterior trunk. Using a single silicon cup with light to medium-strength suction, move the cup laterally on the posterior trunk, starting from the spinal column and moving outwards, towards the front of the abdomen (**Figure 8.40A, B, C, D, E, F**).

Finish off the treatment by covering the patient's back with a hot towel for at least ten minutes.

Cupping massage to the neck:

- relieves neck tension and spasm

- eases stiff neck and shoulders

- helps reduce tension headaches

- encourages blood circulation to the spinal cord

- stimulates the central nervous system

- stimulates the nerves supplying the arms.

Cupping massage to the back:

- improves blood and fluid circulation

- strengthens back muscles and tendons.

Cupping massage to the back of the body:

- stimulates limbs as well as the internal organs, through an intimate association between the cervical (8 pairs) and thoracic (12 pairs) nerves

- improves breathing and the lung capacity

- gets rid of muscular back tension

- improves digestion and helps with the elimination process.

Cupping massage to the lower back:

- helps to reduce menstrual cramps

- brings a sense of relaxation and calm.

A WORD OF CAUTION

- Avoid using glass cups on the lateral muscles (latissimus dorsi muscles) as the ribs are located just below the surface and this area could be sensitive or even painful during cupping massage.

- Cupping massage is possible on a fleshy spinal column. However, avoid cupping directly on the spinal column if the patient is thin or bony.

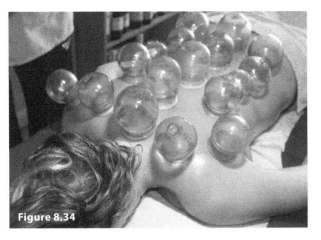
Figure 8.34

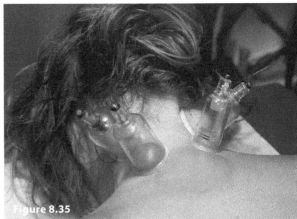
Figure 8.35

This page:
Figure 8.34: Back of the neck
Figure 8.35: Upper back
Figure 8.36: Remove all cups from the upper back
Figure 8.37A, B: Neck massage
Figure 8.38A, B: Shoulders
Facing page:
Figure 8.39A, B, C: Posterior trunk
Figure 8.40A, B, C, D, E, F: Continue
massaging the posterior trunk

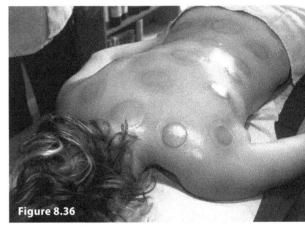
Figure 8.36

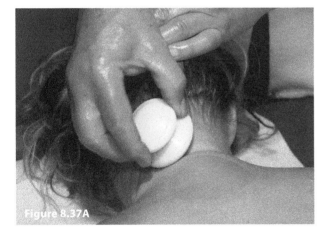
Figure 8.37A

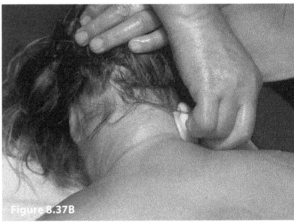
Figure 8.37B

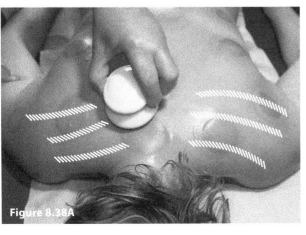
Figure 8.38A

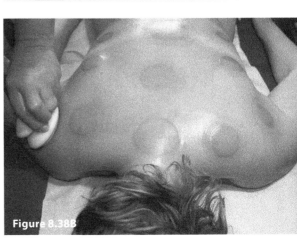
Figure 8.38B

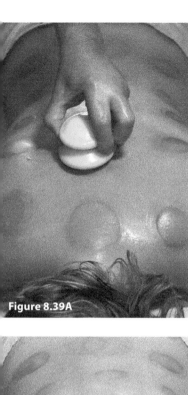

Figure 8.39A

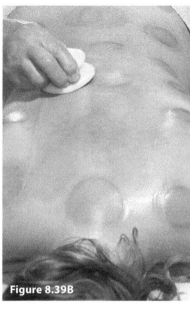

Figure 8.39B

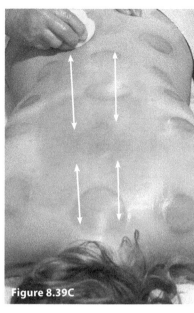

Figure 8.39C

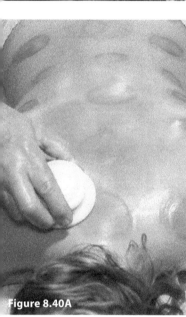

Figure 8.40A

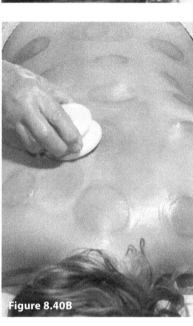

Figure 8.40B

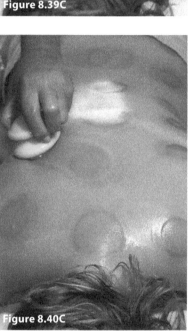

Figure 8.40C

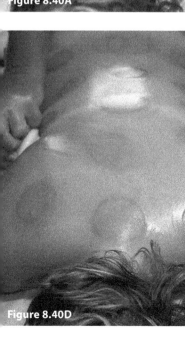

Figure 8.40D

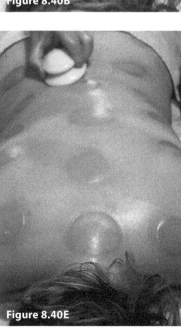

Figure 8.40E

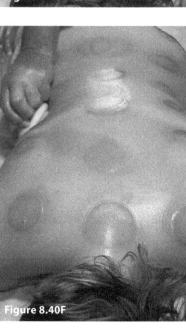

Figure 8.40F

Cupping massage protocol for buttocks and legs

Buttocks

Start the treatment from the buttocks (gluteals) and work inferiorly (downwards) towards the feet. The gluteal muscles which make up the buttocks consist of three muscles: the gluteus maximus, gluteus medius and gluteus minimus. During cupping massage, however, only the gluteus medius and the gluteus maximus are stimulated.

CM 1: Apply massage oil liberally to lubricate the entire treatment area. Apply 10–20 medium-strength static cups on the back of the leg including the buttocks, hamstrings, IT band and calf muscle, for five minutes (**Figure 8.41A, B**).

CM 2: After removing the cups, choose a single rubber or silicon cup (the cup should fit the practitioner's palm comfortably, which helps to maintain full control of the cup throughout the treatment). Follow the contour of the gluteal muscle and move the cup laterally, starting from the base of the spine, over the gluteal muscle and towards the hip. Repeat the same movement five times, each time moving the cup to different position in order to massage the entire buttock (**Figure 8.42A, B, C**).

Iliotibial (IT) band

CM 3: When treatment on the the buttock muscles is completed, move the cup to the outer side of the thigh, on the IT band. Move the cup inferiorly (downwards), applying long strokes reaching the outer knee (patellar ligament) (**Figure 8.43A, B**).

A WORD OF CAUTION

In many people, massaging the IT band can be a painful experience. Applying extra massage oil and light cupping suction can reduce the discomfort.

Hamstrings

CM 4: Massage the hamstring muscles in both directions, starting from the top of the thigh and sliding the cup towards the back of the knee and back towards the buttock (**Figure 8.44A, B**).

Calf muscle (gastrocnemius muscle)

CM 5: Using a small cup, massage the calf muscle by moving the cup from side to side, working towards the Achilles tendon (**Figure 8.45A, B**).

CM 6: Complete the leg massage by applying cupping massage to the entire leg, starting with the calf muscle and working upwards, towards the buttock.

When one side is completed, move to the opposite side and repeat the cupping treatment exactly as above.

Sole of the foot (plantar aspect of the foot)

CM7: Using a pistol-handled cupping set, apply four or five static cups on the plantar aspect of the foot. The sole of the foot can tolerate medium-strength to strong suction and for a longer period of time. According to the principles of reflexology, areas (zones) under the feet are linked to the internal organs. These zones can be used both diagnostically and therapeutically to detect and correct imbalances relating to a particular organ (**Figure 8.46**).

Finish off the treatment by covering both legs with a warm towel for 5–10 minutes.

Cupping massage to the legs and feet:

- improves blood and fluid circulation to the extremities
- reduces fluid retention
- relieves aches and pains
- reduces muscular cramps
- gets rid of tired-leg syndrome
- stimulates lymphatic drainage
- helps reduce cellulite
- brings a sense of relaxation and calm.

Cupping massage on the soles of the feet:

- stimulates the reflexology zones, benefiting the entire body.

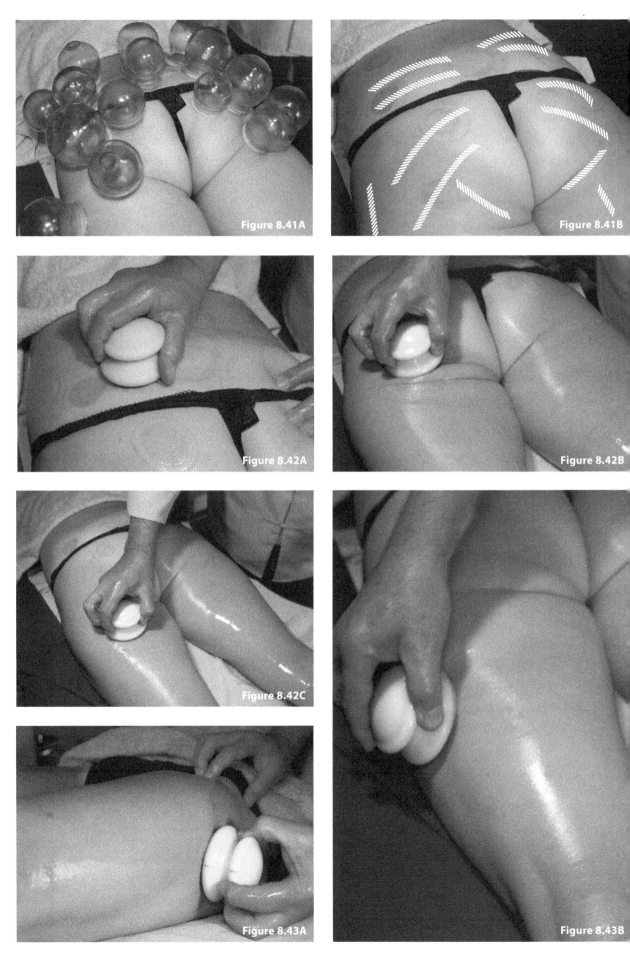

Figure 8.41A

Figure 8.41B

Figure 8.42A

Figure 8.42B

Figure 8.42C

Figure 8.43A

Figure 8.43B

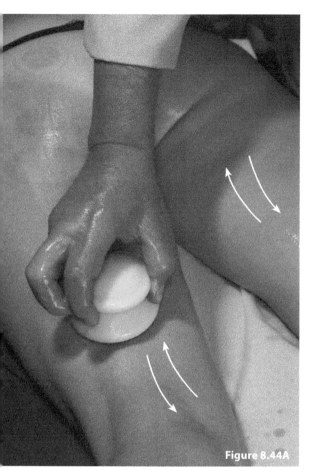

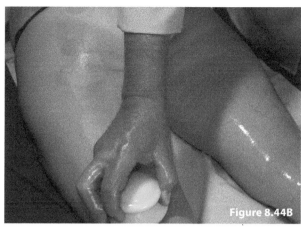

Figure 8.44B

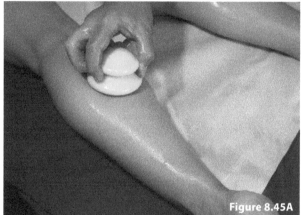

Figure 8.45A

Figure 8.44A

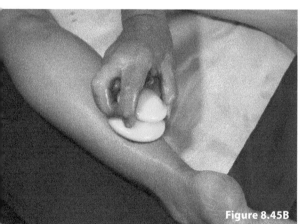

Figure 8.45B

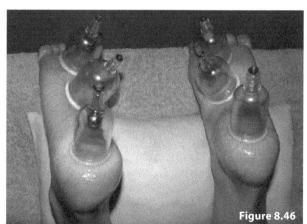

Figure 8.46

Facing page:
Figure 8.41A, B: Buttocks and back of the legs
Figure 8.42A, B, C: Massaging the buttocks
Figure 8.43A, B: Iliotibial (IT) band
This page:
Figure 8.44A, B: Hamstrings
Figure 8.45A, B: Calf muscle (gastrocnemius muscle)
Figure 8.46: Side of the foot

.... • • • ....

CHAPTER 9

SELF-CUPPING MASSAGE

Self-cupping massage is not only convenient but it can also be a very rewarding experience. One of the advantages of self-massage, apart from the obvious financial reward, is that you can actually determine the time that suits you and the frequency, speed and strength of the suction, depending on your mood! Unlike some massage techniques where the actual massage can be done over clothing, cupping massage must be performed directly on bare skin. So, take a moment or two and experiment with light, medium-strength and strong cupping suction on various parts of your body. Discover the tender and the sensitive parts as you do so. You can actually self-administer cupping massage to the entire body except your back. The umbilical-cord cupping set may come handy when trying to get to hard-to-reach parts of the body.

As the massage rule goes, begin with the upper body (face and neck) and work towards the feet. Choose the most appropriate and practical cupping equipment that you feel comfortable with and follow the instructions from the relevant section of the book (**Figures 9.1A, B, C, 9.2A, B, C, D, E, 9.3, 9.4, 9.5, 9.6, 9.7**).

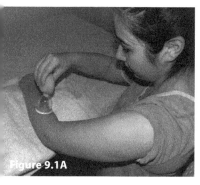

Figure 9.1A

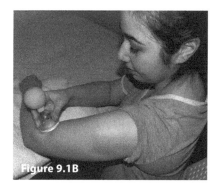

Figure 9.1B

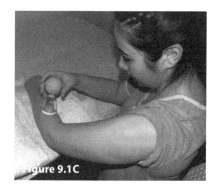

Figure 9.1C

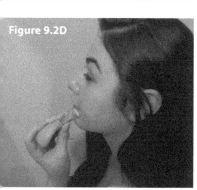

Figure 9.2A

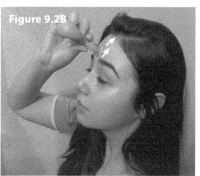

Figure 9.2B

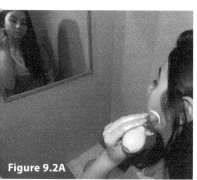

Figure 9.2C

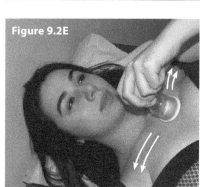

Figure 9.2D

Figure 9.2E

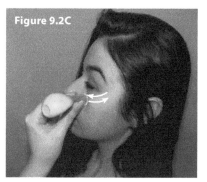

Figure 9.3

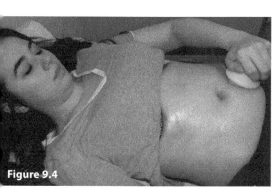

Figure 9.4

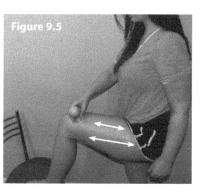

Figure 9.5

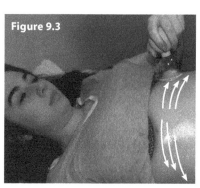

Figure 9.6

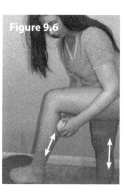

Figure 9.7

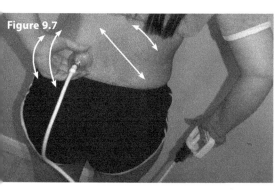

Figure 9.1A, B, C: Arms
Figure 9.2A, B, C, D, E: Face
Figure 9.3: Chest
Figure 9.4: Umbilicus
Figure 9.5: Legs
Figure 9.6: Hamstrings and calves
Figure 9.7: Lower back and buttocks

The first part of the body to be cupped is the arms. You may ask: why start from the arms and not from the face? Starting from your arms will give you the opportunity to practise and develop or improve your cupping skills on your arms, rather than on your face! A sitting-up position, resting your arm on a table or on a stool, is the most convenient and practical position while working on the arms.

As always, before the start of cupping massage, apply oil generously and massage the treatment location first. For easy application, choose a medium or a small silicon cup. With your free hand, press the top of the cup downwards and expel the air so that the cup is secured on the arm. Once the desired suction is obtained, start moving the cup in an up-and-down motion between your elbow and wrist (five cupping movements will be sufficient). Next, move the cup between your elbow and the tip of your shoulder, altering the cup's sliding movement with each stroke, so that the whole arm is massaged. Next, turn to the inside of your forearm and move the cup between your wrist and the inside of your elbow. Complete the arm massage by applying medium-strength to strong cupping on the palm of your hand, this time using a pistol-handled cupping set. Repeat the cupping massage on the other arm.

Facial cupping massage is also best performed while sitting in an upright position, preferably in front of a mirror. By doing so, you can see your skin's reaction to your cupping technique and adjust the strength of the suction accordingly. Follow the facial cupping massage protocol described in Chapter 8 (third eye, forehead, under the eyes, lips, cheeks, chin, under the chin, neck and upper chest).

For cupping massage under the chest and on the diaphragm and the abdomen, the best position is lying on your back. Draw an imaginary midline from the tip of the sternum to the pubic bone. Starting from the top of the abdomen and under the ribcage, move the cup over the diaphragm laterally (outwards), until the cup touches the bed. Work your way down to the lower abdomen and the pubic bone.

From the same position, continue with the umbilical cupping massage. At this stage, additional massage oil might be necessary. Starting from the edge of the umbilicus, move the cup in a circular clockwise motion, expanding the circle with each movement.

Cupping massage of the leg can be performed either from a standing or from a sitting position. Begin from the top of the leg muscle and move the cup towards the knee. Work on the inside of the leg and finish off massaging the IT band.

The back of the legs (hamstrings) and the calf muscle (gastrocnemius) are best massaged while standing and resting the foot on a chair or stool.

The lower back and the buttocks (gluteus maximus) are best massaged while lying on your side.

Detoxification with cupping therapy application

What is detoxification?

The term 'detoxification', or 'detox', is often used to describe a body cleansing process of the internal organs from environmental pollutants such as heavy metals, poisons, pesticides, damaging bacteria, food waste, drugs and alcohol. Our bodies are capable of self-cleansing, but sometimes this self-cleansing mechanism may need intervention in order to do the job efficiently, particularly when we have overloaded our system by over-indulging!

Bodily signs that may indicate the need for a detoxification include:

- unexplained headaches

- feeling tired on waking up

- feeling depressed without obvious reason

- skin complaints, particularly itching, anywhere on the body

- halitosis (bad breath)

- muscle soreness or painful joints

- forgetfulness

- poor concentration.

Our lymphatic system is the main cleansing system for the toxins in our bodies, and the system works through movement. Unlike our blood circulatory system (cardio-vascular system), which relies on the heart muscle to pump oxygen-rich blood around the body cells, the lymphatic system relies on the physical movement of the body parts or the application of cupping massage.

With cupping massage where deep tissue manipulation is possible, one can actually observe the gradual elimination of bodily toxins through the skin! This is made possible by observing the colour of the cupping marks left on the skin. Usually, dark cupping marks indicate high toxicity or a circulation blockage, particularly during the first three visits, gradually fading away (a sign of reduction of toxins) in follow-up visits. This is also an indication of improved blood and fluid circulation, leading to healthier-looking skin. People also report feeling lighter, sleeping better, feeling more energetic, experiencing reduction in muscular pain, and feeling less anxious and more positive!

Detoxification cupping therapy protocol

Before embarking on a cupping therapy detox programme, make sure that the patient is not suffering from constipation and has been regularly emptying their bowels in the past five days. If not, advise the use of herbal laxatives to promote daily emptying of the bowels. Next is the administration of diaphoretic herbs in order to promote perspiration (sweating) and the elimination of free radicals and toxins through stimulation of the skin with cupping therapy.

I normally prescribe my own diaphoretic herbal tincture consisting of at least five herbs (making sure that the patient is not allergic to any of them) and ask the patient to take one teaspoon in 0.5 litre of water three times a day with meals during the detoxification period. Dietary advice includes avoiding the following: sugar in any shape or form, fruit, fried foods, dairy products and red meat. Plenty of high-fibre vegetables, freshly made lentil or vegetable soup, pulses, salads, black or brown rice, fish, free-range eggs, poultry (including turkey) and herbal teas such as burdock, mint, cinnamon, ginger, lemon balm, dandelion, elder and yarrow are recommended during the programme.

Front of the body

Oil the body and apply the rapid cupping technique using 30–40 cups for 15 minutes to the front aspect of the body, covering the chest, abdomen and legs (**Figure 9.8A**). After removing all the cups from the body, employ light moving cupping to the whole of the front and back aspect of the body (**Figure 9.8B**).

Back of the body

Once the front aspect of the body has been treated, ask the patient to lie face down and repeat the same cupping procedure to the back of the body, including the shoulders, back and legs.

(If you are an experienced cupping therapist, use 3–4 glass cups to apply a traditional rapid cupping technique with the fire cupping method (hot cupping); if you are less experienced, the pistol-handled cupping set (cold cupping method) will be equally effective.) This action promotes perspiration and the elimination of toxins through the skin. When this is done, the healthy skin will glow!

Back of the body

Once the front aspect of the body has been treated, ask the patient to lie face down and repeat the same cupping procedure to the back of the body, including the shoulders, back and legs (**Figure 9.9A, B**).

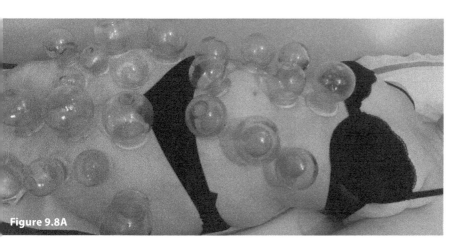

Figure 9.8A

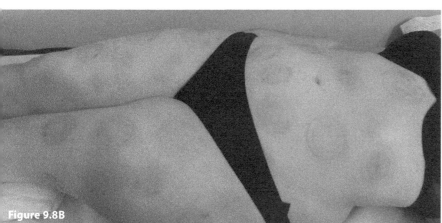

Figure 9.8B

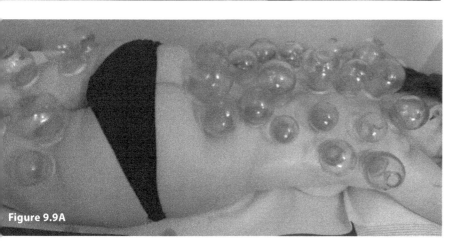

Figure 9.9A

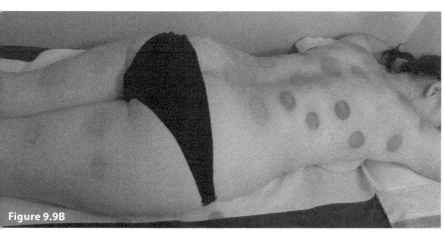

Figure 9.9B

Figure 9.8A, B: Rapid cupping application to the front of the body

Figure 9.9A, B: Rapid cupping application to the back of the body

.... ◆ ◆ ◆ ....

CHAPTER 10

HOW SAFE IS CUPPING THERAPY?

Generally speaking, with the exception of few pathological medical conditions (see below), like any other medical practice when performed by a trained practitioner, cupping therapy is very safe and has no side effects. For more than 35 years in my own clinical practice, I have not witnessed any serious cupping accident or damage. However, that is not to say that it does not happen, especially when the cupping is performed by an unqualified cupping enthusiast!

The most common cupping therapy mishaps are:

- **During dry cupping:** dropping the flame or burning alcohol on bare skin, on clothing or on hair; dark, deep bruises forming on the skin and blisters developing on the cupped location. Dry cupping can safely be performed 1–3 times per week.

- **During wet cupping (bleeding):** excessive bleeding and skin infections are the most often seen adverse situations. Both are indeed serious medical conditions, but, at the same time, conditions that can be avoided entirely. It is not advised to bleed more than once a month.

Side effects, precautions and contraindications

Side effects may include:

- cupping marks or bruises which can last up to three weeks

- temporary light-headedness, feeling dizzy or nausea post-treatment

- fainting (rare) when cupping is performed in a sitting position.

Precaution is necessary:

- when treating people complaining of extreme tiredness or lethargy

- when administering cupping therapy on an empty stomach (i.e. when the patient is fasting)

- during pregnancy (great care is needed for the first six months of pregnancy and should be completely avoided after that)

- when treating patients on anticoagulant medication as this can cause excessive bruising or in some cases prolonged bleeding

- when treating people with sensitive or thin skin

- for patients with hypertension or hypotension

- for patients using topical steroids, which can lead to skin thinning, bruising and enlarged blood vessels

- when treating children: extra care is needed when cupping children; cupping therapy should not be performed on children under the age of four years.

Cupping is contraindicated in the following patient groups:

- people recovering from a recent contusion, angina, cardiac complications or any form of cardiac operation

- those experiencing elevated emotional situations such as a heightened state of anxiety, depression or panic attacks

- patients suffering from high temperature

- patients with skin infection

- those suffering from dehydration or from severe or prolonged diarrhoea

- those with lymphatic cancer conditions

- patients with inflamed organs or whose organs have been perforated – for example, gastric or duodenal ulcers where bleeding is ongoing

- patients with ongoing inflammation such as thrombosis or phlebitis (superficial thrombophlebitis)

- patients with any kind of tumour

- those with blood disorders such as anaemia, haemophilia and other bleeding disorders

- patients with deep vein thrombosis (DVT)

- children under the age of four years.

Cupping should be avoided on the following areas:

- on varicose veins

- on areas of recent trauma such as fractures, cuts or burns

- over bleeding wounds

- over skin moles.

.... • • • ....

CHAPTER 11

FREQUENTLY ASKED QUESTIONS (FAQ)

Is cupping therapy safe?

Yes, all cupping methods described in this book are safe when performed by a trained and competent practitioner who abides by all the precautions listed in Chapter 10.

Does cupping therapy hurt?

Normally, a pulling sensation is experienced on the skin. The pulling sensation (the suction action of the cup) should be well tolerated by the patient. Depending on the individual's skin sensitivity, the power of suction might be too strong for some people, causing pain. This can be avoided by maintaining constant communication with the patient.

Should I bleed from the cupping site?

With the dry cupping technique, sometimes a small amount (a few drops) of blood is drawn out from the treatment site if an acupuncture treatment preceded the cupping application. Otherwise, no bleeding should occur during a dry cupping procedure.

....

Where on the body should cupping treatment be avoided?

Cupping application is not recommended over the eyes and the genital areas.

How long do the cupping marks last?

Normally, faint cupping marks disappear within a week. However, darker cupping marks may last up to 20 days.

How long does each cupping session last?

It is recommended to limit the first cupping session to five-minute intervals for each anatomical location. This can be increased gradually, to up to 30 minutes.

I feel slightly tired and sleepy following cupping treatment. Is this normal?

Yes, due to increased blood and lymphatic circulation, some people may feel light-headed, sleepy or tired following a cupping session.

Can I go to the gym after my cupping treatment?

Generally speaking, vigorous activity immediately after cupping treatment is not recommended. However, I have often applied moving cupping over tight hamstrings before an athletic event, with favourable results.

Can I go for a run following a cupping session?

The answer to this question is an unqualified yes if the cupping is applied to treat an individual muscular complaint. Running should be avoided, however, if the treatment is targeting more constitutional conditions such as tiredness and weakness.

Should I eat before a cupping treatment or have the treatment on an empty stomach?

An empty stomach and a full stomach should both be avoided. It is best to have a light snack an hour before the treatment.

What is the best time of the day to have cupping therapy treatment?

Any time of the day is possible.

Is cupping therapy dangerous when fasting?

Only the dry cupping method is suitable when fasting. I do not recommend the wet cupping technique during the fasting period as this may result in hypotension.

Will cupping therapy interfere with my prescribed medication?

No, cupping therapy will not alter or interfere with the medical properties of any drugs or herbs.

Can I have cupping treatment during menstruation?

Yes, cupping therapy before onset, during or after menstruation is fine.

Can I have a bath after cupping therapy?

Yes.

Does cupping therapy cause any form of skin damage?

No, none of the cupping methods mentioned in this book will cause or result in permanent skin damage. However, as mentioned earlier, temporary blisters or cupping marks can occur and can sometimes last for up to 20 days.

Why do I mark or bruise so quickly after cupping treatment?

Let's make one thing clear: cupping marks are not bruises but can be described as 'ecchymosis'. The *English Medical Dictionary*[1] describes a bruise as a 'contusion or dark painful area on the skin, where blood has escaped under the skin following a blow'. Ecchymosis, on the other hand, describes *painless* discoloration of the skin caused by the local leakage of capillary blood under the skin. All blood-thinning medications, for example, can result in skin ecchymosis. I personally prefer to call these effects 'cupping

---

1   Collin, P.H. (1987) *The English Medical Dictionary*. London: Peter Collin Publishing.

marks'. Given the fact that each individual's skin sensitivity varies, it is quite normal that some people mark more easily than others.

How many cups are usually employed during one session?

Depending on the body part that is being treated, practitioners may use 5–15 cups in one session. In Far Eastern countries, however, it is quite typical to see up to 60 cups used in one session!

I suffer from blocked sinuses, can I have cupping treatment on my face?

The best way to treat blocked sinuses with cupping therapy is to apply moving cupping technique to the local area, using soft cupping equipment with minimum suction.

CHAPTER 12

REALITY AND MYTH

As with so many ancient healing practices, cupping therapy has been the subject of numerous exaggerated claims. First of all, cupping therapy is not magic! The healing process takes time and patience. Cells do not repair and regenerate overnight. The repair mechanism of cells requires the right environment and conditions to perform properly. Cupping therapy's objective is to achieve just that, helping to prepare a suitable healing environment.

Reality

- Cupping therapy promotes blood microcirculation.

- Cupping therapy benefits the lymphatic circulation and drainage.

- Cupping application helps dilate blood vessels.

- Cupping therapy benefits skin by way of improved blood and fluid circulation.

- Cupping application stimulates fibroblasts to produce collagen and elastin.

- Cupping application helps to relax tired muscle mass.

- Cupping therapy assists muscle mass with recovery time.

- Cupping therapy provides deep tissue massage and manipulation.

Myth

- Cupping can make you taller.
- Cupping treats cancer.
- Cupping cures cancer.
- Cupping reduces cholesterol.
- Cupping cures diabetes.